These are stories of hope and resilience, of strength under adversity, of self-reliance and new-found sources of support. They offer one core message to all who suffer from the diverse and difficult manifestations of EDS: You are not alone.

Clair Francomano, MD

Ehlers-Danlos Syndrome is another form of the human body. Just as there are tall people, short people, dark skin colored people, and light skin colored people, each with their own set of medical issues – similarly there are hypermobile people and not so hypermobile people who have different medical issues. Our understanding of EDS has improved, but we still have a lot of work to do. While the medical world works on understanding Ehlers-Danlos Syndrome, people with EDS have provided us with stories of courage and ingenuity. These stories give others and doctors the strength to find solutions.

Pradeep Chopra, MD

As a physical therapist who works with many patients suffering from EDS, I've seen firsthand how isolating and frustrating EDS can be. Along with a more knowledgeable medical field, what these patients need most is an understanding that they are not alone and to be given hope. 'Our Stories of Strength' provides both community and hope and will be just as effective as any medication or exercise.

Christopher Gnip, PT, DPT

Even in the foreword I felt as if I was reading my own story.....it had my attention right away and I went from reading the sample to making the full purchase within minutes. So great to at least know that I am not crazy....well maybe just a little but more appropriately I might have this disease and I can feel validated. Easy to read...and keep reading.

An Amazon Reviewer

our stories of strength

LIVING WITH EDS

Our Stories of Strength
Living with Ehlers-Danlos Syndrome

Edited by:
Kendra Neilsen Myles
Mysti Reutlinger

Foreword by:
Clair Francomano, MD

It is with great hope for better health, positive changes within the healthcare system, financial stability and security, and the ability to balance the daily needs of our children; Jaden, Johann, Seamus, Simon, and Hallen, that we have worked diligently to create this book. This book is dedicated to each of our children. May your future be bright, beautiful, and filled with joy.

Table of Contents

ACKNOWLEDGMENTS

There are many people to thank and acknowledge with regards to developing an idea into this book, and providing support, encouragement, commitment, and more. We want to affirm that this list is likely not complete and is by no means in any particular order.

To all of our family and friends who have encouraged, believed, and supported the importance of this project from idea to inception, we thank you. We know that without your support, the long hours we have invested would have been much more difficult.

Kristi Posival: Thank you from the bottom of our hearts for all your work done on the cover of this book. At each juncture along the way, you have reached beyond the vision we had to deliver a work of art.

Meghan Newsom and Chris West: From idea to inception, the hypermobility photo shoot was incredible. We cannot express our gratitude for your permission to use these photos in the book.

Dr. Francomano: Our gratitude for your support and encouragement for the inspiration provided throughout your work in the EDS community and beautifully expressed within the foreword.

Our sincere appreciation to Pradeep Chopra, MD and Christopher Gnip, PT, DPT for your support, encouragement, and statements to the community.

To the community we have been blessed to be a part of for more than a short time, thank you. We truly are humbled that you have shared your stories with us and allowed us to help you share your voice. We are also grateful for all of you who have reached out to help us share this book, have offered to write, and so much more. Your support means more than words can express.

We cannot say thank you enough for all you've added to this not-so-little book, Carol Schaengold. Your time, knowledge, and insight shaped this collection of stories into a resource and reference for years to come.

Thank you, Laurie Rosenthal Seiler, for your work in designing the logo for Our Stories of Strength™.

We are grateful for the physicians who have believed in our symptoms and opened the door to a better quality of life, as well as supported our efforts to help others find the same within their communities and lives. We are determined to live a life greater than we could have dreamed. You are instrumental in helping us navigate through the ups and downs to achieve all our dreams. Thank you.

Finally, we would like to extend great appreciation to the organizations, Facebook pages, and writers who have shared this project within the Ehlers-Danlos community online. Your excitement and support shown through sharing and encouraging submissions has been incredible. This community is an inspiring collective.

FOREWORD

For many people whose lives have been affected by Ehlers-Danlos Syndrome, the journey is a long and lonely one. Doctors may not recognize or understand the symptoms, schools and employers are often unable or unwilling to accommodate special needs, and often most distressingly, family members may not be able to understand or support their loved ones. Patient support groups such as the Ehlers-Danlos National Foundation are a ray of light in these dark places, providing authoritative information on the many faces of the syndrome and making available resources to allow affected persons to communicate with one another and share information.

While the medical community knows far more about the various manifestations of Ehlers-Danlos Syndrome than it did when I first started practicing medicine in 1980, we still have many questions left unanswered. The good news is that there are now, more than ever, scientists, clinicians and researchers looking into the root causes of those forms of EDS for which the genes are not known, the links between seemingly disparate complications such as dysautonomia and mast cell activation disorder, and ways in which we can best help people with EDS live healthy, pain-free lives.

The stories in this volume are another ray of sunshine for the thousands of people who struggle with the many symptoms of Ehlers-Danlos Syndrome. These are stories of hope and resilience, of strength under adversity, of self-reliance and new-found sources of support. They offer one core message to all who suffer from the diverse and difficult manifestations of EDS: you are not alone.

WRITTEN BY CLAIR A. FRANCOMANO, MD

Director, EDNF Center for Clinical Care and Research Greater Baltimore Medical Center

THE TRENCHES

The most beautiful people we have known are those who have known defeat, known suffering, known struggle, known loss, and have found their way out of those depths. – Elisabeth Kubler-Ross

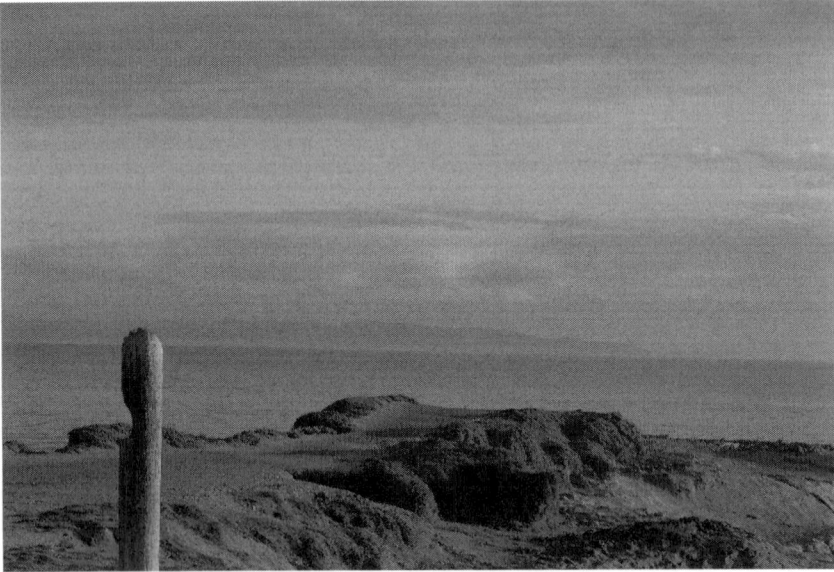

Photo by Gwynne Moore

A Bump on the Head

One afternoon at school, I was playing a game on the playground. I ran and slipped on a stair. I fell and hit my head which split my eye open. I was fine walking until I reached the swings. I collapsed. The next thing I remember was being helped into the school. I don't remember getting to the nurse's office, but remember being in there. I sat for a little bit and talked to the nurse. Then my mom came and picked me up.

My head hurt really badly while we were going to the emergency room. When we got there, my head still hurt, but not as bad as when we were driving. The doctor stopped the bleeding and stitched up the cut. She told me that my head was hurt pretty badly and I could not play in gym or outside for a month. My headache and the ringing in my ears lasted that long, too.

A month after I hit my head, I ate some hummus. I didn't like it. A few minutes later, my throat was burning and I had hives all over my body. My mom gave me medicine and it calmed down a little bit. I saw the doctor the next morning and she said she wanted me to see an allergist and put me on more medicine.

It took two days before the hives were gone and my stomach stopped hurting. My mom sent me back to school when I seemed better. That day, she talked to the nurse because the doctor gave me an EpiPen. The very day I went back to school, I broke out in hives and the nurse called my mom and sent me home. My mom took me back to the doctor who was worried about the additional reaction.

Over the next two weeks, I missed quite a bit of school because I kept having hives and an itchy throat. It was hard to breathe, too. Then I saw the allergist. He talked to me and told me he would do a scratch test. It hurt to lie on the table and have them poke my back. Then it started itching REALLY BAD.

The doctor said I was allergic to many foods and things outside. He put me on a different medicine and asked my mom to take all the foods I reacted to out of my diet for three months. My mom did what she was asked, but I didn't like eating the same foods all the time.

Even though my mom made sure I followed the diet and took the medicine my doctor ordered, I still have severe stomach pain and reactions that needed an EpiPen. I didn't like going to the hospital or having doctors poke me with needles. I didn't like eating and I was scared that I would have another bad reaction.

My mom and dad took me to a hospital we had never been to before when I had another bad stomach pain attack. The doctors did some tests and told us that my reactions were because of Ehlers-Danlos Syndrome and mast cell activation disorder (MCAD). They told us that I should see a doctor in Denver for more tests and that the bump on my head probably triggered the mast cell issues in my body because of the stress.

My mom took me to see the doctor in Denver and the allergist again. The doctor in Denver wanted to see the results of my next skin test and said a biopsy would be best. When I saw the allergist, he tested everything I was allergic to before but this time I didn't react. I only had one spot on my back that was itchy.

We learned that MCAD was common in Ehlers-Danlos Syndrome and we had to learn how to deal with the problems. I have medicine I take that helps keep my body from reacting and I have to eat many different foods so I'm not reacting to whatever I eat most often. Sometimes playing outside causes me to react, too.

This has changed my life because I had to leave school and I can't eat the same foods that most kids do. Sometimes I am sad because of this, but I'm learning how to take care of myself with healthy foods and exercise. I hope that I can go back to school, but I want to learn more about caring for me first.

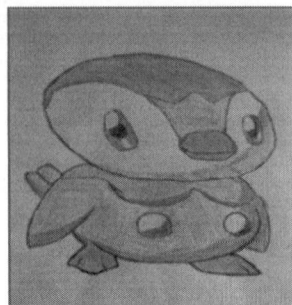

A bump on my head changed my life, but I've learned more about living well since. Sometimes we have to get through the bad stuff to find a better way of living.

AS TOLD BY JAY

Jay, also known as MC DarkMage, is 10 years old and lives with EDS. His hobbies include Minecraft, music, and art. He shares his passions at **MCDarkMage.com**

Good things come to those who believe, better things come to those who are patient, and the best things come to those who don't give up. - Unknown

The Patient Nurse

At 2 years old I was diagnosed with a condition that little was known about called Ehlers-Danlos Syndrome. We knew to monitor for complications and treat troubles as they arose, but there was no cure or medicine to fix it like there is for, say, diabetes or hypertension.

I spent a lot of my earlier life adjusting and hiding my pain. Because there was so little understood about it, my complaints of chronic pains seemed as though they were fake or a child trying to avoid school, so at a certain point I learned to stop complaining. As I've grown, I realized that was a terrible plan. It has led to depression and worsening of certain symptoms and conditions, but when you are a child, you become conditioned to keep quiet.

As I grew into a young adult, my body essentially demanded I acknowledge the condition; the many joint subluxations, disc troubles, migraines, bruising and pain – lots of pain. I've coped, done physical therapy for about every joint in my body, and now wear braces for certain ones such as my ankle and sacroiliac joint. I experienced a blood clot in my leg due to an episode of immobility related to a sacroiliac issue. That resulted in 2 weeks of hospitalization and intense physical therapy. I look back on that time and realize how lucky I am to still be alive. Blood clots are serious business and I could have been far worse off.

I managed to graduate from college with a Bachelor of Science in Nursing and obtained my license as a Registered Nurse. I truly believe that my experiences and all that I deal with help to make me a more compassionate and understanding nurse. Oftentimes, when I tell a patient that I know what they're going through, they are skeptical. I will give them just enough information to understand that I can truly empathize, not just sympathize. Over the past 8 years of my career, I've discovered that a majority of my experience is rooted in my personal trials and tribulations. I'm able to identify a sprain vs. a fracture easily and I can comfortingly explain the process of an MRI or CT scan to a patient. The world of physical therapy is one I can confidently discuss with patients and encourage them to follow through on their ordered treatment.

It's difficult walking both sides of the medical field. In my role as a nurse at a primary care community health center, I see patients with chronic pain, acute pain, and chronic disease. I work to educate, advocate, and manage their conditions. There's a fine line of information you can/should share with a patient – we learn in nursing school to avoid becoming too personal. In my 8 years of experience, I've learned that sometimes divulging a bit of personal information can help a patient to trust you, rely on you, and be honest. These are the most rewarding relationships that I find in my career; a patient who is honest and trusting. If I have to express that I, myself, have back pain problems to help them trust me in managing their back pain, then I will do so.

Being on the other side of the hospital bed, as the patient, is a difficult role for me at times. I can read all of the research, and be up to date with latest treatments in my professional role, yet as a patient I am still in the care of someone else. I've found that having Ehlers-Danlos Syndrome has always presented a fair amount of difficulty for providers. Many don't know what it is… or the complications of it. I've met with so many doctors, that I now call seeing a new doctor an "audition." I view seeing these different providers as my chance to determine if I feel I can trust them to know what they are talking about, be knowledgeable about EDS, and allow me to feel confident in their care.

If there is one major take away I'd say I have from being a patient and a nurse, it is the importance of advocating for yourself. Nurses and doctors and even x-rays and MRIs are still not a perfect science. The human body is a mystery on many levels. You will run into doctors who think they've got the right diagnosis, but if you feel that something else is going on, I urge patients to push for more answers. Get a second or even third opinion if needed. Many of the people I've met with EDS have had to fight to get the diagnosis.

As a nurse, I have certainly experienced difficulty with worsening chronic pain. Bedside care was not something that I could manage for very long and therefore I did not. I sought outpatient care as a safer option for myself. It became clear early on that I would need to disclose my condition to some of my bosses and co-workers as you can only be limping at work for so long before questions start to be asked.

In my current role, my colleagues are incredibly understanding and compassionate. This helps me greatly in my day-to-day struggle. There are always days that I will be at work and it will be evident that I should be at home in bed, resting on ice. I refuse to accept this most times, and I will show up and work with a smile on my face to hide the pain. I would rather this than let EDS stop me, or put me in a wheelchair or worse, prevent me from furthering my career and education.

Chronic pain, at the young age of 29, is not something that is understood well by my peers. At times I may feel like I am an 80 year old, like when things snap, crackle, and pop when I stand or I can't walk for longer than 15 minutes without needing a break. These times, I feel angry and depressed. I want to be able to jump out of bed and decide to go walking around the city for hours. Unfortunately for me, I need to plan my days and schedule my time around my physical ability, medication doses, and doctors' appointments. This can be disheartening, but I know I could always be worse. That is my mantra I suppose: "It could always be worse."

I frequently say "we deal with the cards we are dealt" and accept that this is my life. Not to say that there aren't times when I am angry, sad, frustrated, jealous, bitter, depressed, and even hopeless. I will put on that brave face and smile and be the best actress in the world as I pretend to be "normal." The truth, however, is that it stinks at times and it isn't fair, but we deal with the cards we are dealt and it could always be worse. This is where community is so important. Communicating with people who have had the same experiences and truly understand what it is to have Ehlers-Danlos Syndrome has been paramount to my emotional well-being in recent years. I am grateful that Facebook brought me to a new community of people, living in my city, my state, my region, and my country. Together, we deal with the cards we are dealt.

WRITTEN BY CAITLIN MARTIN

Full time RN, BSN in the Boston area working in the community health arena. Caitlin is struggling with the pitfalls of being chronically ill while learning and striving to become the best patient advocate she can be for herself and those for whom she cares.

I am grateful that Facebook brought me to a new community of people, living in my city, my state, my region, and my country. Together, we deal with the cards we are dealt. -Caitlin Martin

Hope in Living with Vascular EDS

I lost my father at age 45, my brother at age 36, and my son last year at barely age 39. While in the hospital he was genetically tested and found to be EDS Vascular Type IV. I was tested as well since there is a 50% chance of it being passed from parent to child. We suspect that my grandmother had this genetic disorder. My grandparents on both sides are from Russia.

Both my son and I were diagnosed with Gene: COL3A1, Mutation: TG576 Chromosome #2 mutated on position 1727 substituted G to A. We were told that we have a variant that has never been identified - Variant at PG576D.

I have bruised (like a person on prednisone) and torn my skin easily all my life but it had gotten worse as the years have progressed. I am 64 years young and still going! Amazing since I was told that average life expectancy is around 40. Upon speculation, I believe that my grandmother passed this on since she lived to into her late 70s as did my father's father. All the men in my family have died from complications of arteries and intestines failing.

I am 5 feet 1 inch and weigh 101 pounds & my husband (a chiropractor/acupuncturist), (thank goodness) suggested that I start taking large doses of buffered, time-released Vitamin C (to bowel tolerance) along with Rutin every day. I am on 11,000 mg of C a day and if I miss one day of taking it I start bruising (black bruises) and my skin begins tearing again. I have been on this dose (twice a day) for several years and it is the only thing we know of that helps connective tissue. I have to believe that this has helped me.

Oh - one other piece of info is that even though my blood pressure is good my cardiologist put me on the smallest dose of Norvasc in order to keep my veins and arteries at the same constant pressure.

Hope you all enjoy each and every day as special and live your life with a passion!

WRITTEN BY CAROLE HIBNER

From the Editor: As we learned more about Carole, we couldn't have been more inspired by her story as she finds a way to live her life with passion. She lives with Vascular EDS and is currently 64 years young. The information she included in her story below is not meant to serve as a prescription for treatment. If you are interested in her tools in the toolbox, please schedule an appointment with your physician and discuss what is best for your particular case.

Zebra Art

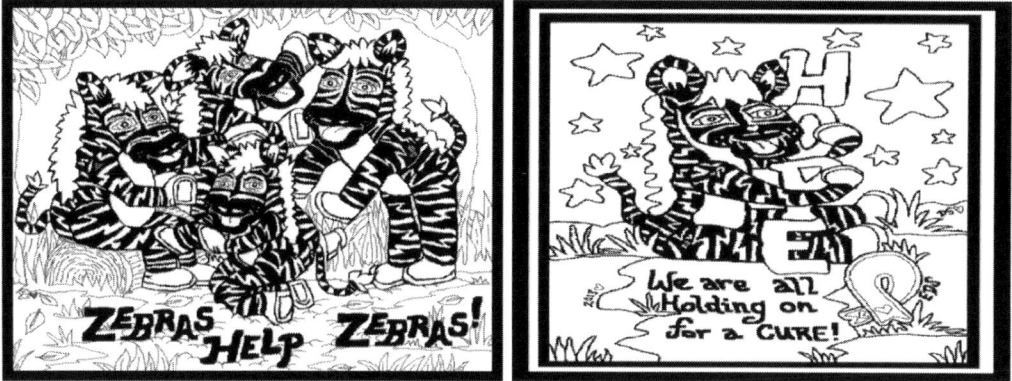

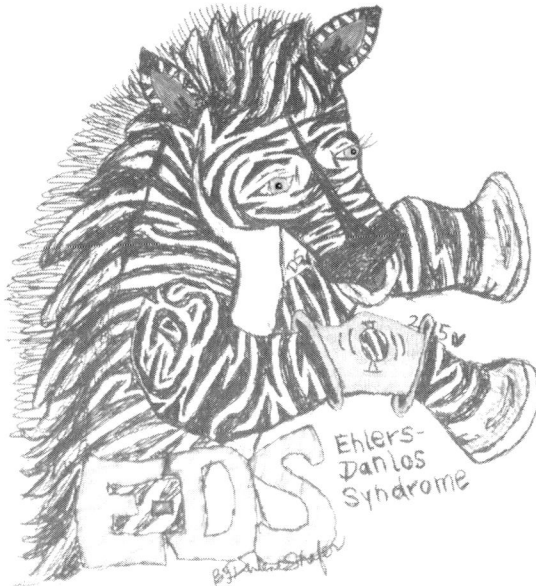

Drawings by DarWcWizard

*Life only comes around once, so do whatever makes
you happy, and be whomever makes you smile.*
– Unknown

My Name is Rachel

This is the story of me.

My body is full of surprises, as you will soon see.
I have strange joints, not just my elbows and knees.
I can twist and turn my arm completely around.
Make my elbow point up and my hand point down.

When I walk down the hall my knees make loud noise
Reminiscent of a bowl of crunchy cereal or rattly toys!
This might not be odd if I was 60 years old
But I am 14 and my joints shouldn't be quite that bold.

I have always been bendy and it used to be fun -
I could dislocate a finger and people would run.
But in the last few years it has started to hurt.
Screeches and howls – I just might blurt!

I am weak and dizzy at the drop of a hat.
I would fall to the floor when chasing my cat.
My weakness got worse and in stepped chest pain.
Our doctor was stumped in the diagnosis game.

My momma was worried and didn't know what to do.
I hate her phrase "What AM I going to do with you?"
Doctors and specialists and hours of research,
POTS was decided, yet it got worse.

I look like a poster child for some horrible disease,
When I run a fever, have a migraine, and sneeze.
There weren't any triggers that were easy to find,
I'd be sitting on the sofa – lost in my own little mind.

Suddenly I start itching and feel like throwing a fit!
Again, we and the doctors had to research it -
For weeks and months of allergy study time,
Another thing – MCAD – was added to the line.

What does this mean for a girl of fourteen?
It means I stay home, rarely to be seen.
I left my school because I am too weak to attend.
I learn on-line and have to message my friends.

I dislocate my shoulder by walking down the hall.

I tower over everyone because my genes make me tall.
I can't go out in summer because the heat makes me weak.
I stay inside for winter because my fingers burn, white and pink.

Not from the cold that you feel in December
Or even the chill that starts in November.
I struggle in early October just by going to school
And for a 14-year old girl that just isn't cool.

Does this mean I am depressed and hate my life?
Or am I one of a kind, waiting for my knight?
A doctor to fix me and make me well,
So this story is one others won't tell.

I am all about research and spreading the word
So that others like me can have a voice to be heard.
If you have a story that's anything like mine.
Please check my illnesses through these websites online.

No matter what's wrong please reach out.
That is what blogs and support groups are about.
Loving each other, sharing, and support when we can
Even when necessary lending an ear or a hand.

It doesn't matter what you battle day in and day out
There is support somewhere if only you reach out.
Stay strong and remember no matter what you do
There is someone out there fighting just like you.

WRITTEN BY RACHEL VANMETER

Rachel is a 14-year old who lives with her mom, step-dad, brother, sister, four cats, and one dog. She loves to read, write stories, listen to music, and hang out with friends.

Through Their Eyes

I am exhausted. I'm not talking about a bad night of sleep tired, but three-days and nights of flu tired. All the time. With fatigue, I am plagued with pain. It's never a question of if I will feel this way, but how bad will it be today? This week? This month? Dealing with the pain is merely hour-by-hour.

Coping with all of this and attempting to work and care for my family is daunting. I have a 5-year old with EDS like myself. My youngest child is 2. He is absolutely adorable and has more energy than I can keep up with. It was during one of these challenging days that my oldest son asked if I would play with him. I yearned to play so badly, but this pain – it rules everything. Discouraged, I had to say no. I started crying. I was overcome with the feeling that I was constantly letting my kids and family down. I felt so useless, like I was in the way.

It was in that moment that my oldest son walked up to me and gave me a big, gentle hug. As his arms wrapped around me, he said, "Mommy we love you. We don't love your body or your pain, but we love you."

Their love makes living a little more bearable.

WRITTEN BY KERRIE EDWARDS

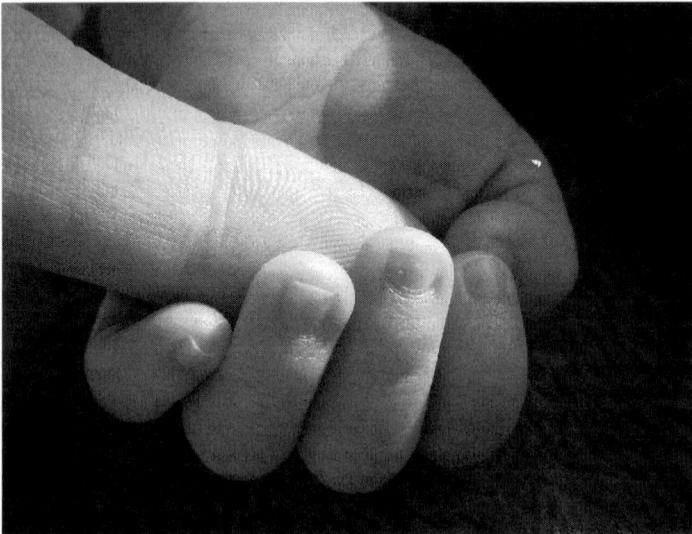

There is No Finish Line

The coldness of the early December rain began to freeze my hands into a clenched fist without feeling. I forgot my gloves.

Why am I walking in the lightlessness of the night, with streaming beads of rainwater falling in seemingly aimless directions off my protective winter gear? (The pain of today's movement shields me from the pain of non-movement tomorrow.) This is my life – life as I've known it since 1993. I must keep moving. I must always keep moving and move no matter the pain it may cause in the moment, nor its later pain or paradoxical relief.

"Agony. Exhausted. I can't. I can't, I… must…"

Flutters of faintly whispered words echoing a hollowed mind pass by me, almost through me, leaving a ghost-like print.

It feels like I am walking on stilts. Each corner of my being throbs. I box this inner dialogue daily. Every motion is calculated enough so professionally, that the casual observer cannot see. Most often, so are my thoughts.

NOT bringing gloves is NOT a smart thing to do when one has Reynaud's, a condition connected to Ehlers-Danlos Syndrome. I have hypermobility type and periodontal type of EDS, and an undefined mutation not specified from my geneticist. I have been "labeled" severe and I know at this age of 46, I am. I have been "labeled" so many things, as Zebras often are, while in process of finding clarity, or while searching for diagnosis or treatments, I sometimes question what I believe.

I have heard far worse stories than my own.

Now, as it was, ten or twenty years ago, if I miss more than a few weeks of regular daily exercise, heading into missing a month of exercise, I WILL become bedridden and have to crawl my way back to standing. I must be regimented, rigid, a regular at the gym and as responsible for my health as I can possibly be within reason. Regular daily exercise for me to maintain mobility is 2½ to 3 hours a day since I was in my mid-twenties. A short or skimpy session would be 1½ hours. I am now standing an hour a day if I am lucky.

I cannot prove this to you, nor do I need to at this point in my life. Some disbelieve me and will stop reading. Others will continue on… one letter at a time. One breath, one curl, one lap, one calf stretch at a time – because that has been the drive of the Zebra in full strut anyway. We sometimes are left to figure out what works best for us on our own device; searching for our disease's name like a one-in-a-million online lover who turns out to be the real thing. I happen to have both, and more. Another fellow Zebra may not need such intensity through exercise to keep them glued together to survive, others may need nothing or little at all. What would that be like? Is that EDS?

But, I do. I DO need up to three hours a day of working out to survive if not more… and I AM standing here now in the rain, like a junkie who has fallen off the exercise wagon. I was in my zone for some time, coming back stronger than ever… I had a hero's welcome before – and now – I see the tsunami coming.

On this December night, the rain is beating a cold, steady stream bouncing lightly off my jacket hood. I focus on my alignment while lifting one foot up, visualizing healthy muscles working in sync as the other foot lands. I begin to picture my gait length and watch if my foot pronates too much in any direction. I am in the dark. No one is around me. I have crossed the street and can see the lights within my home. I will use them as guides, since no streetlights are ever lit here. The sidewalk is empty. I close my eyes and begin to breathe into my diaphragm, big balloon-like breaths to relax myself. I continue to breathe diaphragmatically into each muscle group, starting from my feet and working my way up to the neck, arms, hands and head relaxing and letting go; moment by moment. Twenty-two years now of this meditation that is walking, sitting, standing, and lying has offered me a safe haven of acceptance where the world of medicine and society has often not. Training myself, I cocoon into creating a force field like wonder woman breathing out the pain, and within each inhale I visualize what sprain, what subluxation, what rotated vertebra is out and exhale the pain – cycling a rhythm to put my mind into another space of focus. This is part of Mindfulness Meditation I began in '93. I simultaneously ask what self-help tasks I must do to accomplish the current and most pressing injuries, because, there are always multiple injuries - with varying degrees of urgency. You know this. You juggle. You know this if you live the life of a Zebra Warrior.

In the dark, I begin my secret but familiar limp, which, for all safe purposes, is why I like walking in it. Everyone needs a safe place. It's where I have gathered my thoughts and like with tweezers, dissected the insanity of the paradox. "Don't move too much, you will injure yourself, don't move enough you will become bedridden." No one true professional can truly answer or guide this for me, nor will they ever. If left to their collective advice, I would not write this story. The sharpness of the evening air keeps the incandescent light from dulling my scent such as natural instincts exterminated but yet fed from PUBMED journal reading can often do.

When I am walking and hurried… the keen observer only can spot me in the hunt. I have mastered my illusion for many, and I know it's for their comfort as well as mine. It is here, in this natural sanctity I can really visualize my body as whole, without ailments or pain and practice walking straight, with a Pilates bridge, and then no one can really see me limping as I mentally melt my spasms of the day as much as I can. It's great for the migraine I have had for five months now, too. In the gym or on the treadmill, I can't cry in pain. Nature has never once done a double take. These maple trees, these beautiful trees I am surrounded by, the river, the corn fields and barns I dodge in-between, and I thank them in my goofy, but genuine tree-hugger fashion, soak up my tears. In their welcoming silence I can hear myself and feel my form.

The wave is now pulling back.

Winds gust through me cutting my wet gear as I bury my hands into my sweater to elude the glove-less frozen rain. I see my home from a distance now. I've been walking back to it as I have been in meditation. I need to make a move and cross the street. I can't keep walking in the dark and the cold. I see the light inside my home.

"MY BODY HAS CHANGED!!! I DIDN'T WANT TO DO THIS AGAIN! WHY?!" I lean against a two-hundred year old Maple, staring at my grey colonial protecting myself from the rain. I am now 46 facing serious surgery potential. I ask to a familiar Higher Power whom I reason with, wrestle with, yell at in my mind, speak to in silence, and cry to in a hollowed aloneness sometimes fighting back. I seemingly am comforted by my conversations, as I was enraged with in the same volume of respect. "Why? WHY??? I give back the quarter at the store. I say nothing when I get a dirty look when I need to use a placard because I don't look sick, but hold a door open when for an elderly lady when I am able. I don't lie. I …"

I … I need neck surgery… I told my cold fists to warm my tearing face and stumble, almost falling in grief while making a path in the unmarked snow toward my home. I see the kitchen table with piles of unfinished business.

WE are faced daily with a choice.

I just thought I was done. Cancer, Lyme disease, back surgery, disc herniation, fibromyalgia, and the twenty-year quest for the name of Ehlers Danlos. I thought the name would leave me done…

There once was a sign in the YMCA I saw in my 20s that read, "'THERE IS NO FINISH LINE."

I approach the front door of my home and choose to go in. Tomorrow, I will find my gloves.

WRITTEN BY MONICA CYRAN

Monica Cyran was first diagnosed in 2010. She has been trying to test out for her Master's in Psychology, but has had a few EDS bumps in the road. Although she has completed all of her required hours and course work, she just needs that test! It is her goal to complete this very personal journey and obtain her degree. Monica uses mindfulness meditation daily in sitting, standing, walking practice since 1993 and uses it as a guide to everyday well-being. She incorporates it in pain reduction and exercise routines.

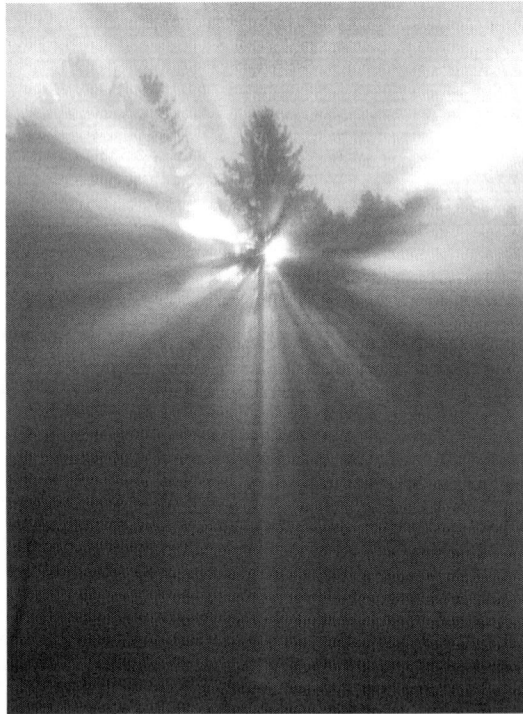

Hear Me

I wish at times you were a spot or a broken leg then people could clearly see what's wrong.
But, no… you are invisible instead.

How can I explain you when people only act upon what they see?
How can I carry this pain that never sleeps within me?

I wish each day that you would disappear or just give me a break.
If not, then be visible, so they would know I'm not a fake.

It's hard to live each day and at times I feel alone
Dragging you through or asking God to take me home.

But, no, I will not let you win as I've been given life to live,
If not for me then for others to understand exactly what it is.

There are many things in life that are hard to comprehend,
Like the TV and mobile phones – and the invisible transmissions they send.

Yes, things are hard to understand and are not always before your eyes...
I ask you to stop and think a while, as it might be an invisible illness in disguise.

WRITTEN BY JULIE R M CHESTERS

When we lose one of our senses, we gain strength in another. – Unknown

Living the Zebra Dream

Since a young child, I've always played many sports.

When I graduated from high school, I started training twice a week in field hockey and played a game on the weekends. I also went to the gym or went bike riding on the days I was not involved in team practice. I was starting to really improve and was promoted to the next team.

At that point, I started having a lot of trouble with my knees. It was really frustrating, as I love playing sports. I lived and breathed sports.

In my second year of university, I had to see a knee surgeon, as my knees were getting worse. At my first appointment with the surgeon, I was diagnosed with hypermobility syndrome, which I thought was nothing concerning. I thought I had been over training. How wrong was I!

There were hours of physiotherapy, icing, exercises to do at home, bracing and taping my knee, regular reviews with my knee surgeon, and closely monitoring my training and match load. We decided that I required surgery at the end of the hockey season. I was devastated! The operation went well and I had a slow, but steady recovery.

While recovering, my left knee was getting worse. A decision was made to have the same procedure on my left knee in July 1997. Unfortunately, the surgery didn't work as well. Three months after the surgery I was still in a lot of pain and had much instability.

I consulted my knee surgeon again and he agreed that something wasn't right. More scans were ordered and a second opinion was sought. At the end of my university year my surgeon decided to operate on my left knee again to stabilize my kneecap. It was the best decision, although it did take a long time to recover from, as my quads were very weak from being on crutches for a year.

During that year I had many counseling appointments with a sports psychologist, as I was so distraught not being able to play sports. It was like my life and soul had been taken away from me. Even though I struggled, I never gave up the dream of playing hockey again. For a while, I was the team manager, but it became too much watching them. I decided I needed to find some new interests.

I started doing some voluntary work for the Australia-Japan Society of Victoria. My main responsibilities included contributing to management decisions for the Committee of Management, coordinate the subcommittee for Young Members Group, and organize events for the Kanpai Club, a young professionals group. Other roles included attending the National Conference of Australia-Japan

Societies held in Cowra, NSW in August 2001 and participating in a ten-day business study tour sponsored by the Japanese Ministry of Foreign Affairs in March 2001.

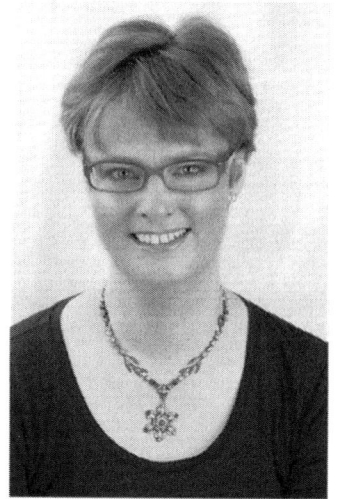

Although I was staying active, it was one of the most distressing times of my life. My friends were off having fun and enjoying their lives and I wanted nothing less for myself. The world felt dark.

There are many different shades of color along this journey. Some dark and lonely with others bright and surrounded by loved ones. The dark hues of surgery, depression, and my dreams fading away blend with the bright colors from the support of family, friends, surgeons, physicians and therapists. Together they weave the scarf of my journey.

For quite a few years my knees seemed to be quite good. So much so that I moved to the UK on a working holiday and was then granted a work permit for a permanent job working for a global wine company, which I really enjoyed. It took a lot of courage and strength to move away from my support networks, but it was something that I had always wanted to do. It was one of the best decisions I made. It changed me as a person. I gained confidence and a love to travel.

While working and living in the UK I had the opportunity to travel to France, Germany, Croatia, Scotland, Ireland and many parts of the UK. It was a dream come true.

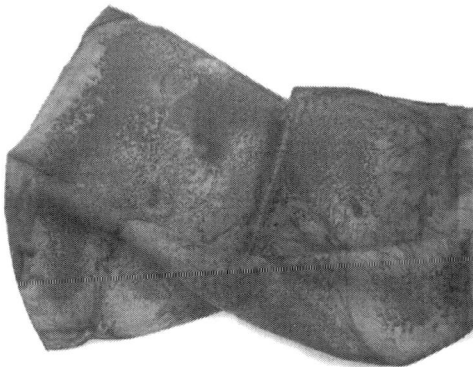

After coming back from the UK, I started having a lot of problems with both knees dislocating and subluxing medially. I had a number of soft tissue operations, but none of these seemed to work very well. In 2007 and 2008 I was involved in two car accidents, neither were my fault. The instability in my knees worsened, requiring additional knee surgeries between 2008 and 2011. It was absolutely devastating. I never thought I would get through it all.

Although I am still not where I want to be in my health, I have found something that keeps me going – silk painting. I can sit down with a silk scarf and disappear from the struggles. I can put the stress of daily life behind me while I focus on the act of painting.

Silk painting gives me a positive means to enjoy my time when I might not be feeling my best. Living with Ehlers-Danlos Syndrome has many ups and downs. It means we need to be inventive with the type of work we do, evaluate the way we do the activities we love, and decide which outings are best for us on any given day. We also need to work with our support team to decide which treatments will work best. This allows each of us to still have a very fulfilling life.

WRITTEN BY KIRSTY WILKINSON

Your attitude is like a box of crayons that color your world. Constantly color your picture grey, and your picture will always be bleak. Try adding some bright colors to the picture by including humor, and your picture begins to lighten up. – Allen Klein

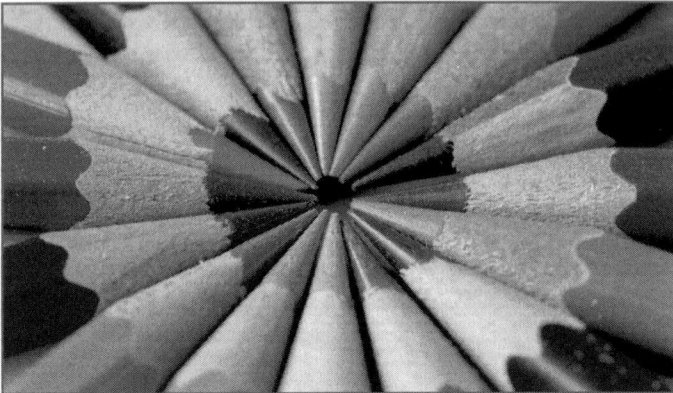

A Hodgepodge Life

The alarm went off after I was already awake for the day. I turned it off and sighed, "It's going to be a doozy. Thank God my head feels like it's sitting well." I grabbed a cup of coffee and turned on my computer. It was 4 am -- time to get working.

Early mornings and I are friends, comrades. It's the brief few hours of peace and quiet that allows me to work diligently before the chaos of parenting, homeschooling, phone calls, text messages, and emails beg for my attention. I cherish these early mornings in ways I never thought I would. They are also the time where I assess my health and shift to-do's around to accommodate how I feel. Some mornings all I can do is curl up with a book and stay still.

I've been through much, but this life is mine to accomplish my dreams.

The early start seemed as though it wasn't early enough. I ran into hiccups with sites not propagated, themes not quite working correctly, and information missing. As I sorted through the issues in succession, I heard the laughter signaling my time in the office was through. I packed up my laptop and moved to the living room just in time to see my children come out of their room.

"What's for breakfast today?" Oh, yeah. I should eat, too. Smoothies or fruit? "Fruit leather and applesauce."

"Can we watch TV this morning?" No, it's Thursday. We have school.

"I don't know where my big book is, Mom." Have you checked in your room, on the bookshelf, or on the table? It might be there.

"What is this word?" Allegiance. "What does that mean?" How about you look in the dictionary?

"Can I work on the letter C today?" Of course. Cat, cab, catcher, coat, car... "Oh! I want to draw a car."

Meanwhile the phone rings for the first time, right on cue. 9 am. Before answering, I ask my oldest to read to the youngest while I take the call away from the chaos. Ten minutes later we are onto math. This continues for another hour before all the necessary courses are complete.

We need to move. Let's walk around. "But I don't want to!" We must. It will help with your back pain. "Fine. Can we see the fields?" Sure.

An hour later and we've walked all along the dirt roads by the fields. We spotted some horses and pregnant cows.

Horses – I need to find that quote from Dr. Heidi Collins about horses of a different color.

"Can we watch TV now?" For a while, then you both need to draw or play outside. "Yay!"

I move the chair and sit at the table again to work. Where was I? Oh yes… I need to send a few messages out about this project.

The morning quickly turned to afternoon and more calls, messages, and work were completed. I might just tackle this list before dinner! It was about that time when I heard a ding that caught my eye – a message on Twitter from a business owner I have been meaning to touch base with again. No more delays, I thought as I responded, "If you are available, I could call or you could call me."

A few minutes later, the phone rang. We talked as though we were old friends catching up on life, health, and work. As questions were asked, I walked and talked, scoring another mile to my day. Proposal by Monday? Perfect. I'll be working all weekend on a couple of projects.

"Is there anything I can eat?" You'll have dinner soon. Your brother is cooking tonight. "Okay."

As I stand writing notes and quotes from the call I was just on, there's a tug at my pants. "Mom, I have this funny rash. It's on my legs, too." I look him over from top to bottom. Are you breathing okay? Is your throat tight? "I'm breathing fine and my throat doesn't feel itchy." I'll get you some medicine before you eat. Let's watch this until then. "Okay."

I have Ehlers-Danlos Syndrome, but it doesn't have me.

I stand back in awe at the day that transpired. Normal, routine, and perfectly mine. There were plenty of hiccups and challenges along the way, but what is normal for us isn't normal for everyone. I'm a Mom living with EDS and raising two boys who inherited this crazy condition from me. We don't stress or panic over allergic reactions, pain, or fatigue. We just keep plugging away at the lists of tasks and moments we wish to experience. It's nothing spectacular, but it's spectacularly ours.

I work hard to teach them now how to care for their bodies with diet and exercise. We deal with the chaos just like everyone else, but for me – I have hope. I hope that each of my children will be strong in their 30's – never having to drop everything to focus on regaining their health, doctors who will be well educated in how their connective tissues make for strange occurrences, and they will remember these days from childhood where their Mom looked disability in the face and told it to shove off as she built successful businesses from the ground up so she could balance both their needs and hers without being defined by Ehlers-Danlos Syndrome.

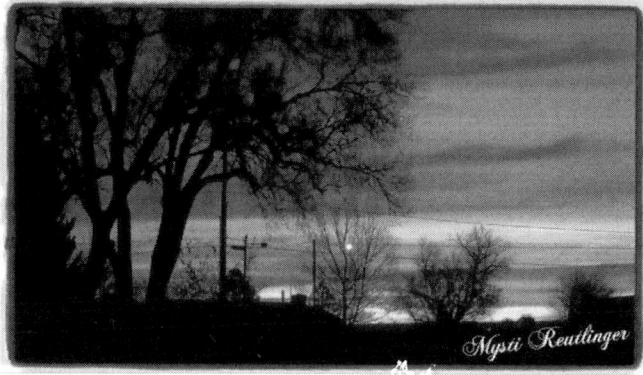

WRITTEN BY MYSTI REUTLINGER

Mysti Reutlinger is the author of *Journey to Health: A Holistic Approach to Ehlers-Danlos Syndrome*, *The Pantry Cleaner: Chemical Free Cleaning*, and *A Gratitude Journal for Grieving Parents*. She is co-owner of Our SOS Media, LLC, works with parents who have lost a child learn how to embrace life again, encourages parents of preemies to advocate for their children, and jumps at the opportunity to speak and educate physicians on Ehlers-Danlos Syndrome all while raising two boys she teaches to cherish each day.

Connect with Mysti on Twitter **@MystiReutlinger** or Facebook at **Mysti Guymon-Reutlinger**.

> *Love myself I do. Not everything, but I love the good as well as the bad. I love my crazy lifestyle and I love my hard discipline. I love my freedom of speech and the way my eyes get dark when I am tried. I love that I have learned to trust people with my heart, even if it will become broken. I am proud of everything that I am and will become.*
> *– Johnny Weir*

Just 5 Minutes

It's a rainy Thursday morning and I've just sat down at my desk to tackle some work. I'm staring at my computer, not knowing where to start or how to begin. I'm exhausted, in pain, scared and feeling defeated. I don't like feeling defeated. Defeated isn't me or who I am or what I stand for, so I have to find a way to feel strong, get my feelings out and move on. So, I'm sitting here writing, not really knowing what will come out. I have a headache, a cervical migraine to be exact, that started last night and was caused by sitting too long working on my computer. So, why am I sitting here again? I don't know, other than I have so much work to do, feel incredibly overwhelmed, scared, worried, have phone calls to make, bills to pay, emails to return, appointments to make, various things I've committed to people, have to be at the school for my 6- year old's class birthday party at 3 pm and my husband is away again. And the reality is, I just don't know what else to do right now. "Brain Fog?" That's an affirmative.

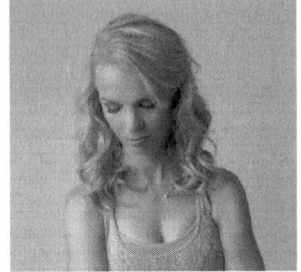

I'm struggling for sure, but this is all part of the roller coaster that I always talk about. I know this roller coaster well enough to recognize when fear and anxiety are getting the best of me. And that combination, along with a horrible headache, fatigue and chronic pain, isn't the best combo for me or for anyone. When this happens, I know enough to go to my "safe" place of just finding a way to meditate; to quiet my mind and do what feels right at that moment. I don't answer the phone, check or respond to emails, look or post on social media, clean, or work, and I try to forget about my never-ending "to do" list, countless bills that must be paid, the blog posts I want to write, and the various ways to bring in additional money. I turn off all sounds other than ones that are calming and just <u>be</u>. Sometimes, my safe place is writing, reading, listening to calming music, reading, watching something mindless, practicing "normal" meditation, moving or stretching my body in some way, or, according to my husband and kids, hiding in the bathroom by the heat vent. It is times like this that I have to remind myself to focus on what I CAN do and control; even if it seems like nothing. I have to quiet my mind, trust and believe that things will get done, I will figure "it" out, and things will be ok.

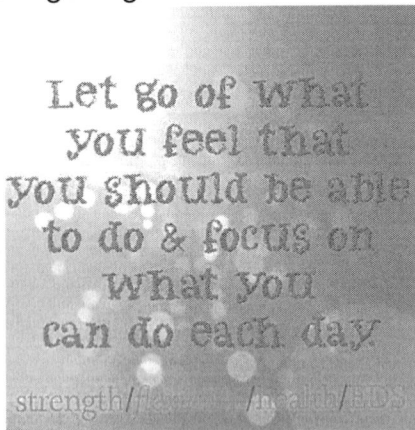

Let go of what you feel that you should be able to do & focus on what you can do each day

strength/ / /health/

So, here I am... meditating while writing, because I desire to help people by sharing information that I have, but I recognize that I am human and fighting the same fight as those I want to help. We all need to know that we aren't alone in our struggles – and that people **do** understand. That's my hope in writing this...

that there are people who understand what I'm going through in this moment in my life. I'm not alone in this struggle and neither are they.

My struggle this morning began last night after working all day at my computer. I had to face the stress of our financial situation, the near-constant worry, sleep deprivation, pain from not moving enough, and my brain overloaded with ideas, plans, and hopes to make our situation better. I could feel the headache coming on, my husband helped me as best as he knows how and rubbed my temple and the base of my skull so that I could go to sleep without getting sick to my stomach. I did sleep, but woke up in the middle of the night with the usual ache in my hips, shoulders, and neck. The headache was still persisting and I prayed that it would be gone by the morning. It wasn't. My husband got the kids ready and took two of three to school to help ease the burden on me knowing this headache still persisted. He made the boys' lunches so I wouldn't forget, because I forget often; all of the time, really.

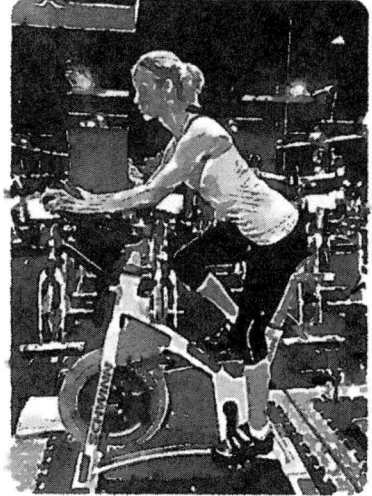

Yes, there has been pain and hurt. But now I choose to be free in this moment. – Unknown

I wanted to scream. I feel awful and sick to my stomach. I'm scared. How am I going to take care of the kids when I feel so terrible? I don't want them to see me this way. Please help me keep this away from them. But… I can't do that.

My husband is trying so hard to support us and he worries about me constantly. I need to be strong for him, for the kids, and for me. This morning, I snuggled my babies as I lay in bed trying to appear tired, but happy as usual, while pressing on just the right spot on my head that would help alleviate the pain in my neck and above my eye. My husband kissed me on the forehead and told me that he missed me already and left. My oldest ran out the door with him to his math class, I yelled to make sure he heard me say goodbye. Then I prayed to myself, to God, or to whomever in the universe would listen.

"I pray that we make it through the last 2 months of this math class. Then I will let the school know how I really feel about this advanced math class for 4th graders… This class that is part of the curriculum and is appropriate for my son and he deserves to be taught math at his level, however, this class is early in the morning, before elementary school even starts and it's at the middle school. I'm not sure anyone considered how "walkers" would get to the middle school or maybe they thought that parents of 9 and 10 year olds would allow their to kids walk by themselves at 7:15 am to the middle school?

If they only knew what disruption this class has caused for our little family. Originally, I thought it was only on Tuesday mornings. We've had to choose between our son getting the appropriate math instruction and things like, being able to ride his bike to school with his best friend who is moving at the end of the school year, or walk with his little brother who was so excited to go to school with his big brother. This class is only offered during the 1st period of middle school, which is 1 hour and 15 minutes earlier than when elementary school starts. We even have to have to wake him up each morning, when he really shouldn't have to be up so early. He is 10 years old and is not middle or high school yet! This class is part of the elementary school curriculum, but it is not offered during elementary school hours. We have to wake our younger kids up and schlep them out the door, because our oldest can't walk to the middle school alone and there is no transportation or buddy system for these elementary school kids who are within walking distance to the middle school. Our son likes this class, wants to be in it and is doing well. He deserves to be in a math class at his level. I still ask why, if this is part of the curriculum, is it at the middle school and before elementary school starts? Do they understand how long of a day that is for a 10 year old? He's exhausted, we all are. This class has just tipped us over the edge. A logical guess is that we were already teetering on the edge for the last 4 years and had finally started making strides in stability and routine. Now this… My son deserves to participate in this math class no matter my issues.

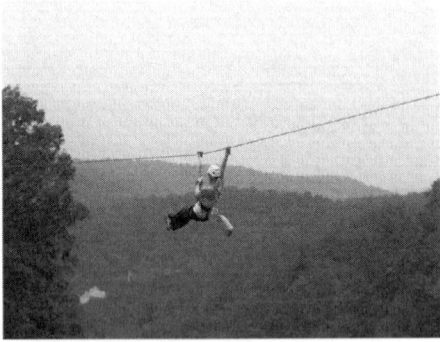

What are my issues anyway? Fatigue, exhaustion, and chronic pain. I'm floundering to keep from drowning. My issue is that because of this class, it takes 3 hours to get three kids ready and off to school – and there's no way to consolidate time. Even the before-care program at the elementary school had a bus to take our son to the middle school.

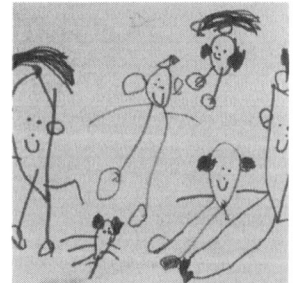

What working parent(s), with no additional help, can take up to 3 hours each morning to get their kids ready and off to school? That's our issue and not the school's. The other option would be for our son to not be in this class that is appropriate for his level and ability. We have dealt with the disruption to our lives, initially believing it would be once a week, but once we figured out that it was every day… the logistics were a nightmare. When the school determined that they could not help us get him there, he had already been in class for nearly three weeks and was doing well. I was even told by someone at the school that I just needed to suck it up and suffer, because that's what she did in order for her child to attend a charter school. My point? Hers was an elective

decision and not one that was based on how the school was going to offer classes associated with its curriculum.

When you are writing the story of your life, don't let anyone else hold the pen. - Unknown

God, give me the strength to release my anger, frustration, and angst with this class. I need to let it go and use this energy for good.

The truth? My issues are from living with Ehlers-Danlos Syndrome. I've done a damn good job at keeping my issues under wraps. I've made a point to show my kids the good that I've done through having EDS like volunteering with EDNF, people I have been able to help, deciding to work for myself instead of accepting disability, and the anthology that I'm putting together with my new business partner. My children do not see how I suffer… Even my husband, who knows about the daily struggles, doesn't know all of it. It's too painful, too raw, and too scary… even for me.

She made broken look beautiful and strong look invincible. She walked with the Universe on her shoulders and made it look like a pair of wings. – Unknown

I like my little bubble and focusing on helping others, because that's where I find strength to keep going. That's why this stupid math class makes me so upset, because it's not as simple as just taking my son out of it. (Stupid … I said "stupid" and we don't say "stupid" in our house.) Again, what would be the reason? The reason would be because of my physical inability to keep up with life. I just can't do that. I won't do it. (I just said "can't" and we don't say "can't" in our family.)

My husband has to travel. He has to do his job and we cannot hire help or constantly ask family for help. There isn't anyone to carpool. This class has just tipped us over the edge and it makes me angry. I shouldn't be angry, because I want what's best for my son and he likes and does well in the class. I have to keep going.

God, why does this class bother me so? Is it the class or everything else that we are trying to manage? At what point do you sacrifice what is best for your child versus what is best for you? This class has made me face Ehlers-Danlos Syndrome, chronic fatigue syndrome, mast cell activation issues, chronic pelvic pain, fibromyalgia, chronic neurological issues, hypothyroidism, chronic headaches, and more each and every day. This class pushes me to the limits – limits I cannot hide. I don't know how to contain it. I must work, I must pay bills… current and the ones that are overdue, I have to handle household tasks… and I need rest, sleep, and a break from my brain to just know that we will be ok.

Isn't 4 years of dealing with crisis after crisis enough for anyone, especially for a family to endure? We've paid our dues, we've trudged through the mud, and we've come out together… still holding on. We've faced financial disaster, job loss, the reality of divorcing or not, a major health crisis, and we still have to find ways to keep up; despite income instability. We've been down the spiral and crawled our way back out. We've hit rock bottom and then some in many ways. We are clinging to what we have left and focusing on our blessings.

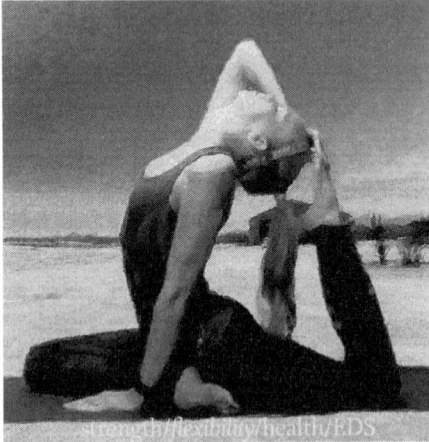

I don't want to take medications to feel better or to keep me going. I shouldn't have to do that. I haven't had to in the past, but now I do. Why? The reality is… in order to help support my husband, his job, and our family, I have to stay up late working because that's when I can do it without interruptions, when I can think clearly and calmly, and find the focus to get through each day, this week, this month, and the next 6 months. I also workout late because I have to care for me, but staying up late makes me tired in the mornings… I hate being tired in the mornings around my babies. (Hate it. I said "hate" and we don't say "hate" in our house). It has to change, but how?

If only our children knew how far we've come, what I've been working on, how hard mommy and daddy are working to support them. We have worked hard to keep our little family together. This is just temporary, at least, that's the only way I can think about it. Being tired in the mornings is normal for me or any working mom with three kids, but it's just been worse lately. It will get better. It has to get better. Hard work always pays off, right?

A great attitude becomes a great day which becomes a great month which becomes a great year which becomes a great life. – Mandy Hale

God, please… don't let me start getting sick. I can't get sick. If I do, I must keep going. I can't go to the ER. I have three kids to care for, my husband has to do his job and has to travel, and I have no back-up support. I can't show weakness or say I have a headache. Everyone has headaches… I have them all of the time. I need to suck it up because I have to pick up the kids later.

I want them to know how much I cherish them and feel how happy I am when they are around me; when we are together as a family, because that's all that matters. I need to focus on not allowing my stress to give them any sense that I am worried about how we will make it through next month and if we are going to have to move, because despite how much mommy and daddy are working, our jobs don't pay us overtime. Sales is feast or famine and when you've had one crisis after another, it isn't always the best job to help provide stability or a means to catch-up. We just can't seem to catch-up. I didn't think it could get worse, but it has.

I worry about what they think of me lying in bed in the mornings. I've been working so much and am exhausted lately. I worry about all of them feeling the same way I felt as a kid with a mom who was always too tired and lying down whenever she wasn't working. I'm not always lying down though… I'm up and active. <u>This is all just temporary</u>. If they only knew what mommy is trying to accomplish, how I'm trying to help ease the burden of supporting the family for daddy, and that our little family is still intact after the four years we've been through… It is a miracle. It's a blessing and the best gift we could give them.

When I stopped telling myself "I will never…." and started focusing on doing something for "just 5 minutes," little by little things began to change.

I am still going to the school for the class birthday party today and I will work out. I have to clean the house, do the laundry, run errands, dishes, make phone calls, prepare taxes, sign up for activities, and pay bills. Ugh … pay bills.

God… I just don't know what more I can do to help change the trajectory of this path that we've been on. When will we find reprieve? What more can I do? I'm not sure, because I am doing more than one person can physically handle. I'm scared, really scared, because I've exhausted all my options or all that I know. God, this is exactly when I miss my mom the most. This is when I want to run to her for a hug and have her tell me that everything will be ok. It really doesn't matter how old you are, you still need your mommy to make you feel better, even just a little.

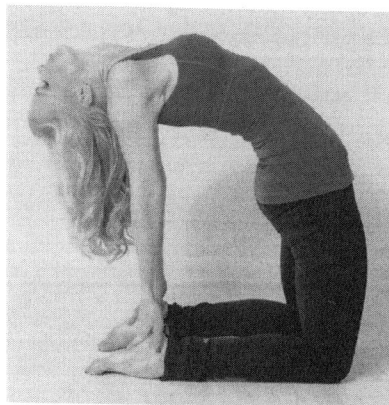

God, if there are more options, please give me a sign. I'm open and willing to work even more. I did medical studies in college for money. I'm not afraid of hard work or working more. I'm not too proud to do things that may seem below my experience and qualifications. I'm strong enough to keep going, even if it causes me more health issues. I can take it, if it helps find stability for my family and helps ease the burden on my husband.

If you can't fly then run, if you can't run, then walk, if you can't walk then crawl, but whatever you do, you have to keep moving forward. – Martin Luther King Jr.

Please, I pray that you help me find ways to support my family and to make it through the last few months of this math class; that the teachers give my kids a break if they are tired, are late or miss school, if writing hurts their hands, if they can't sit still for too long or seem distracted, if they need to go to the health room because their stomach hurts or they have a headache, if homework is sometimes late, or if they have to buy lunch because I forgot to bring their lunches… again.

I pray that teachers, neighbors, and strangers feel empathy when they see toys thrown around our lawn and not picked-up or our garage door left open overnight. The reality is that we had dinner as a family, because that is the least we can do every day, we put the kids to bed, and both Brian and I went on to do more work. We simply forgot about cleaning up the yard and didn't get to it before we finally crashed that night.

I often wish that I could just scream from the top of my lungs, "We are fighting this fight and barely keeping up!" In truth, I've really never felt the need to publicly display my struggles or for others to understand. Nor have I desired to "keep up with the Jones'" – evident by my post-workout, unshowered, still in gym clothes, and no make-up appearance.

Would I like to be put together each day, house always perfectly organized and lawn immaculate? Yes, because to the core of who I am, I am totally OCD, not because I need to be that way for anyone else but myself, because that is what makes me feel good and in control. I learned long ago to let things go, especially when I have bigger fish to fry like kids to feed, time to step away from the rat-race of life, and coping with the roller coaster of living with chronic conditions.

> *I am too positive to be doubtful, too optimistic to be fearful,*
> *and too determined to be defeated. – Unknown*

A simple nod of the head with empathy that silently says, "Hey, I get it. I understand. You are doing the best you can. Your kids are loved, your family is intact, and you are taking care of yourself. That is what matters." In essence, I pray that those who may see those outwards signs of "disheveledness" and lack of "having it together," offer kind words such as, "How are you doing?" instead of "Are you ok? Because you look really thin."

I pray for guidance to continue on through my own journey so that I can use my strengths to help others and help support my family. I pray for understanding and communication between my husband and me, that my kids know how much I love them and see that I'm working hard for them. Please let them not see how tired I seem and stop their worry for me. I pray for my kids' health and happiness and that we may find the other side of this huge never-ending mountain. I must have faith that good things come to good people and hard work pays off. I have to trust you, because that's all we have left and that is what we believe.

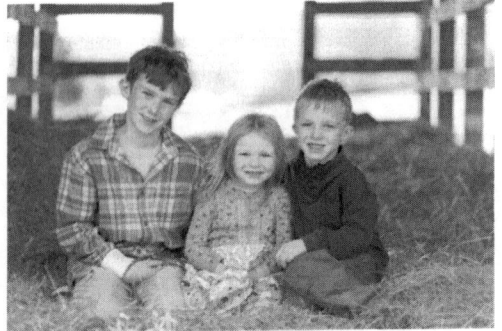

Please, I pray that my feelings about this math class are one day heard and understood, so the next mom who is dealing with similar struggles isn't pushed to have her own difficult yet contained issues spread wide-open for her children to see just because she is doing what is best for her child. That decision, doing what is best for your child, is sometimes enough

to rip-open "MamaStrong" stitches covered with super glue that keep her body and soul together. Amen."

There's only so much a little family can take and so many resources they can pull from. There isn't always more money available to "fix" the struggles and make it all better. At that point, all you have left to cling to is faith, hope, trust, determination to persevere, and strength to keep going – even if it's for just five minutes at a time.

WRITTEN BY KENDRA NEILSEN MYLES

To learn more about Kendra, visit About Kendra Neilsen Myles on page 202

The photos included with this story are a compilation of photos of Kendra, a drawing done by her youngest child, and quotes that hold significant meaning for her.

Professional photographs by Helen John Photography. HelenJohnPhotography.com

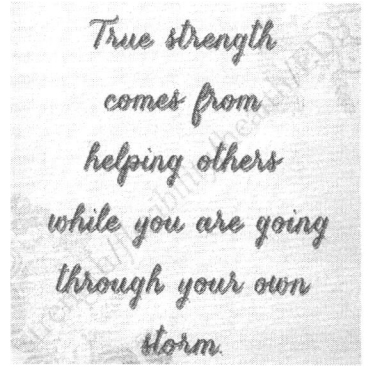

True strength comes from helping others while you are going through your own storm.

CHANGE

You must take personal responsibility. You cannot change the circumstances, the seasons, or the wind, but you can change yourself. That is something you have charge of. – Jim Rohn

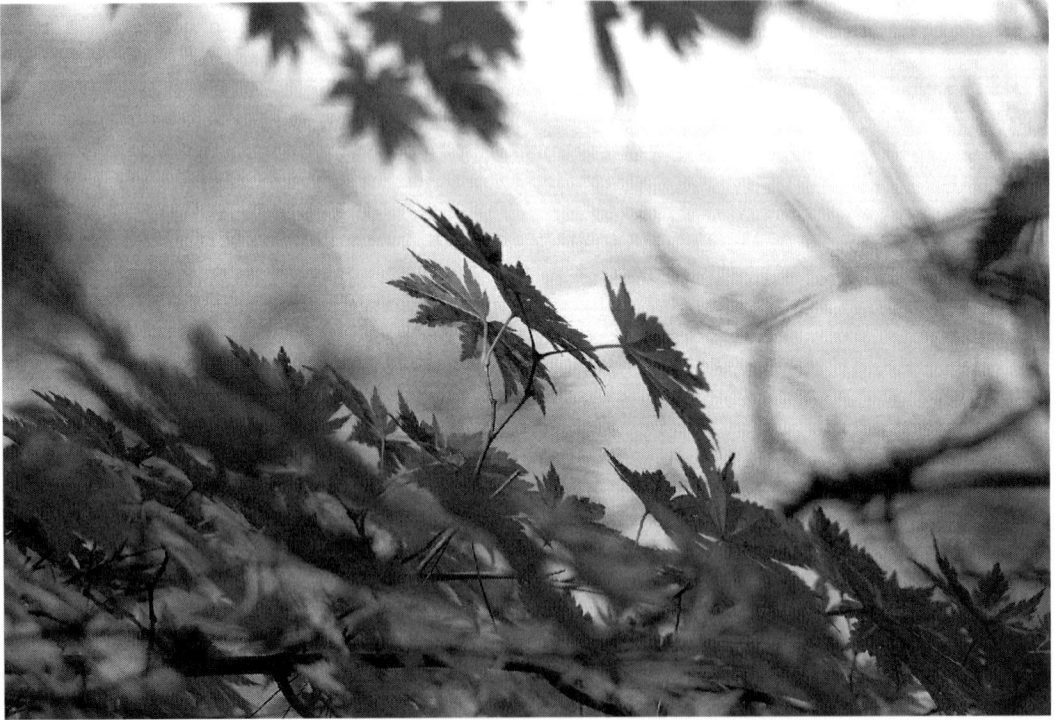

The Warrior's Song

As I sit here, mindlessly putting my shoulder back in its socket, I hadn't even realized it was dislocated. I'm so used to the extreme hypermobility and the excruciating pain that comes with it that I hardly even think about it anymore. Or rather, I can't think about it. I have to keep going... I have to keep moving...

I was diagnosed with Ehlers-Danlos Syndrome when I was a preteen. The doctors originally thought I had arthritis, but after many appointments and a visit to a geneticist, the truth was revealed. My parents didn't know much more than I was "stretchy" and in pain. There weren't enough resources at the time for them to truly understand what I was going through. So I tried to hide it. My skin was so bruised and torn that I would wear long sleeves, even in the summer, to cover up what appeared to be abuse, but in reality it was just my EDS. As the years passed, I went through school, became certified in the dental field, and got a job. I loved my job, but my boss and my coworkers didn't understand my condition. I was called names, and became the center of many jokes. I was exhausted from trying to keep up with everyone and my health rapidly declined. After about a year, I was in the worst shape of my life. I was constantly missing work, I could barely eat, I couldn't sleep due to pain, and my eyelids would swell up so much I couldn't open them fully, and my skin was literally peeling off for no apparent reason. I was only 20 years old, but I felt like I was 120. I eventually had to quit my job.

After a couple more years of suffering, I decided to take my life back. I knew that I could never be cured, but I made up my mind that I was not going to sit back and watch myself rot away. I went on a strict diet, not to lose weight, but to just eat clean and pure. Then I started looking for low impact exercises. I didn't have a pool, and classes that involved dancing around were not a good fit for my wobbly knees and ankles. I tried yoga, but I was too flexible, and injured myself by hyperextending. Then, one day, I came across the art of Tai Chi. It sparked my interest and I joined a class. I saw a huge difference within the first month, in just little daily tasks. I was able to take a shower, do TWO loads of laundry, AND unload the dishwasher, IN THE SAME DAY! I could have cried in happiness. I was able to practice my piano for more than 10 minutes! After playing the piano for 21 years, and having to limit my practice to a few minutes every couple of weeks, I was able to play for two hours in one day.

One good thing about music, when it hits you, you feel no pain. – Bob Marley

Today I feel like a new person. I will never be cured, nor will I ever be completely without pain, but I've discovered that there is hope for people with Ehlers-Danlos Syndrome. A hope that you will be able to walk without a cane, that you will be able to cope with each new day, and that a long life can be lived not spent in bed unable to move. I'm not alone in this battle, and neither are you! I am a Zebra warrior and I will continue to fight to raise awareness and to spread the hope to those who feel so alone.

WRITTEN BY CORTNEY TOUMAYAN

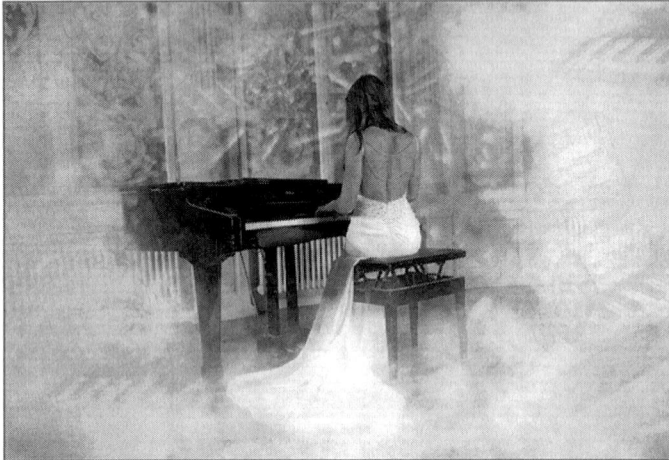

At the end of the day, the only questions I will ask myself are: Did I love enough? Did I laugh enough? Did I make a difference?

5 Tips for Living with EDS

I've had hypermobile joints my whole life. I was told so by a medical professional for the first time when I was 15, after my patella got stuck behind my femur, in full flexion, requiring general anesthesia to relocate it. The orthopedic surgeon explained that I could be a bodybuilder, and without his surgery, I would dislocate again for the rest of my life. I declined. It took me years to rebuild my strength, but I did it. I was more prone to injury than most of my peers, whether in work, as a Licensed Massage Therapist, or in play, hiking, climbing, road cycling, dancing, etc. But I took my body's tendency for injury and used what I learned to teach my clients, and myself about alignment and biomechanics. I am thrilled that I spent more than a decade of my life working with doctors, physical therapists and chiropractors, sharing clients and collaborating on how to help people recover from and prevent future injury. The knowledge and visceral understanding of anatomy has been crucial to how I maintain my health with EDS.

I am the administrator for two online EDS Communities. A member asked for support recently, in regards to how to keep a positive attitude in the face of life changing complications from chronic conditions, and how to keep doing the things you love. Here are some of my tools:

1. Honesty. I have to be honest with myself about what I can and can't do. And those change daily, so it's constantly experimenting and retooling my activity. One week I may function almost like a normal body, and the next I am severely affected and am disabled. Being honest about how my body is doing keeps me making well-informed choices, and avoiding injury as best I can, while also staying active at things I love. I also say be honest about your feelings. Have a good cry, and then get up and focus on what you CAN do.

2. Can do vs. can't. There are a ton of things I can't do anymore. If I stay focused on that I'm miserable, and miserable to be around. Keeping my focus and training on what I can do, and how to modify to keep at it is key for me. Example: my endurance currently blows; so I do multiple short sessions during the day to get the total workout in that I want.

3. Pacing. Not just your workout or weekly social events, I mean pace your workload. I was a Licensed Massage Therapist, for 11 years. I specialized in deep tissue manipulation, injury rehabilitation and chronic pain management. I loved it and I was damned good, too. I haven't worked in over 18 months I still have clients calling to see if I'm back to work yet because they can't find anybody they like as well. At my peak, I could do 15 to 18 hours per week. As I aged and EDS got bigger, I could only do 8 to 10 a week or I was injured and couldn't recover between shifts. For the past 3 years, I did 12 to 15 hours of massage a week, plus other work, well over what I knew was good for me, because I was a single parent and had bills to pay. I ran myself into the ground and am now in a rehab/rebuild state myself. If I had respected my body's limits, and taken it easier in my workload, I am confident I would not have lost my career and identity. Pacing, and working with our bodies can keep us active and healthy for the long haul.

4. Make friends with your body. There is a lot of "I hate my body" and "I hate (insert disease or disorder here)" kind of talk out there. For me, that way of approaching this whole thing is self-defeating because I was literally making my own body, my enemy. Viewing my body as an ally, and at times wounded ally, makes it easier to find out how to do what I want, and I feel better about myself in the process.

5. Gratitude. I know this may seem cliché, but in addition to Mindfulness and other meditation practices, I make a practice of gratitude. I make myself identify all the good stuff in my life that I am thankful for, that I am proud of, that make me smile or laugh, and I do it at least 15 minutes every day. It makes a huge difference in my mood and my ability to see possibilities for treatment and training.

WRITTEN BY JUSTINE CASE

Silent Desperation No More

Until my rare disease was diagnosed, doctors treated me with suspicion when I sought help for my debilitating, but invisible, pain.

After a lifetime of seemingly unrelated physical complaints and inexplicable pains that kept worsening, I was finally diagnosed with Ehlers-Danlos Syndrome at the age of 55. EDS is a genetic flaw that causes the production of defective connective tissue. Weak tissues stretch or tear, body parts aren't held together properly, and joints shift or dislocate spontaneously, resulting in chronic pain and many other health problems.

During my forties, the pain and exhaustion from my still undiagnosed EDS worsened significantly. Sitting at a computer all day at work was straining joints and muscles in my lower back, and even exercising didn't help anymore. The daily pain was distracting me from my work, so I began my futile quest for a medical solution.

I went from one doctor to another and tried every suggested test, procedure, treatment, and therapy, but no one could figure out why I was in so much pain in so many places. Eventually, my neurologist prescribed me opiates so that I could control my pain well enough to continue working and remain active.

By the time I stumbled into my fifties, my life was becoming unmanageable. My ever-increasing pain and fatigue took more and more activities and options from my life; I could barely function at work, and finally I couldn't do that anymore either, even with pain medication.

Until my pain became too disruptive, I enjoyed a successful high-tech career. I worked in the competitive IT field and spent my free time on outdoor activities. I was an endurance athlete who voluntarily suffered frequent injuries and serious pain from extreme physical activities. I rode horses in 50-mile trail races, ran off-road half-marathons in the hills, and annually bicycled four to six 100-mile daylong events in the steep coastal hills. I had always been proud of how tough I was, but eventually the persistent and debilitating pain overwhelmed me.

After twelve years of opiate pain management my doctor retired, and the next neurologist I found had drastically different beliefs about opiates: she didn't want me to take them at all "because they weren't good for me." One after another, I optimistically pursued her alternate ideas for finding and treating the cause of my pain, but nothing worked.

When she couldn't find a cause for my pain, she started to question its existence. She began to doubt my honesty and repeatedly pressured me stop taking opiates. But when I finally gave in and cut back, my pain increased accordingly, both in intensity and frequency, and interfered with every aspect of my life. After a few months of this, life no longer seemed worth living. I lost hope and became desperate, depressed, and suicidal until the intervention of a therapist convinced me to try again.

Before my diagnosis of EDS was known, and without visible symptoms of pain, most doctors simply did not believe the symptoms I reported. When I was accused of imagining my own pain just so I could get drugs, my confusion and distress almost pushed me over the edge.

Many doctors tend to overlook or minimize their patients' pain, and they rarely mention the damage caused by chronic pain itself. I was told opiates are bad for me, yet these same doctors never told me about the accumulating damage to my nervous system from letting my pain continue uncontrolled. While I was taking less opiate medication, I was able to do only a fraction of my previous activity and I spent week after week lying down most of the day.

My pain worsened as I lost the physical conditioning I had struggled to maintain. My muscles were no longer compensating for loose joints, so any weight-bearing movement irritated nerves and triggered muscle spasms. Without opiates, I knew I couldn't control the pain once it started, so I became reluctant to initiate any activity at all. I was housebound, depressed, and increasingly fearful of untreated pain.

Eventually I sought out a more sympathetic doctor, who now prescribes enough opiate medication to make my life bearable. While opiates don't eradicate my pain, they dull it enough to make it tolerable. Now I'm able to get out of the house and get some exercise, and I'm only on the couch a few hours a day. With my body and mind active again, I can manage my remaining pain well enough to find some enjoyment in life, be less of a burden on my loved ones, and contribute to society again.

While doctors and the public are bombarded with sensational media stories of addiction, I want to speak out and give a voice to the untold numbers of people suffering their pain in silent desperation. My mission is to refute the picture of "chronic whiners getting addicted to narcotics" and show how opiate medications can save people who suffer from chronic pain and from the depression, hopelessness, and complete disability caused by untreated pain.

WRITTEN BY ZYP CZYK

Until I was finally disabled by chronic pain and fatigue from EDS and fibromyalgia in 2008, I was a high-tech IT maven at Apple and Yahoo. I live in a small cabin in the redwood forests of the Santa Cruz Mountains "up the street" from Silicon Valley with my husband and various four-legged kids.

Most of my time and energy are devoted to my research and info blog, **EDSInfo.wordpress.com**, which is an archive of the latest science, news, and information related to chronic pain, EDS, and fibromyalgia, plus some of my own writing.

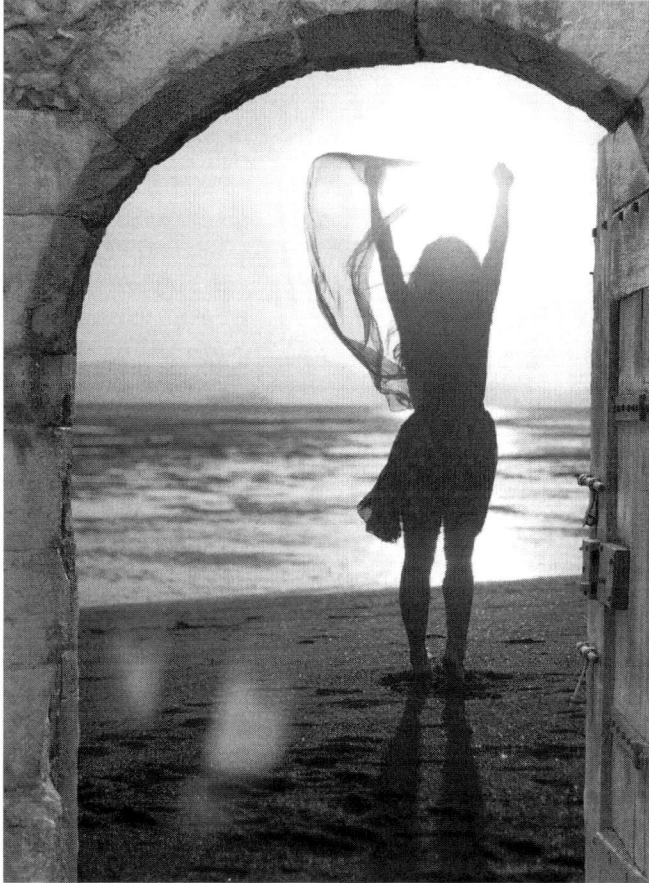

Disabled

Our family seemed to be plagued with one illness after another for many years. We had the sudden death of my grandmother, my young daughter becoming very ill, my sister with severe issues, my mom facing big challenges, and I was always feeling miserable. All of us fighting similar, but different health problems, caused my mom and me to research extensively online. One day we came across Dr. Diana Driscoll's website (**prettyill.com**), who is an Ehlers-Danlos Syndrome patient herself and a huge advocate. Everything clicked; we had Ehlers-Danlos Syndrome with many comorbid conditions! It felt like we were reading our combined medical nightmares word by word and watching it through many of the video posts Dr. Driscoll had on her site. Each problem that we thought was not connected was indeed connected by our faulty connective tissue. I was in disbelief that out of all of the specialists I had seen over many years that not a single one picked up on this connective tissue disorder. It had been overlooked my entire life, 25 years, many spent suffering! It brought mixed emotions of relief, sadness, happiness and anger.

I continued to research long and hard until I finally came up with a plan of action for not only myself but for my family. We immediately got in contact with Dr. Diana Driscoll who gave us so much hope and offered to have my mother participate in a study where we would receive immediate information and treatment to take to our local specialists. My mother was on a flight to Texas within 2 weeks! We finally knew we were not alone and were referred to local geneticist to get clinically diagnosed with EDS. We wanted more answers than we had, though. This was our life and the original geneticists that diagnosed us couldn't provide us with much hope. By God's grace huge things were in the making for the Ehlers-Danlos community! A top EDS geneticist, Dr. Clair Francomano at Greater Baltimore Medical Center, was teaming up with EDNF to open the first Ehlers-Danlos Clinic less than 90 miles from my home outside of the Baltimore/DC area! When I called to schedule an appointment, I was disappointed that it would be 18 months later! I set the appointment, but felt that there was no way I could handle suffering like this for another year and a half.

Defeated and determined, I continued researching. This is when I stumbled upon *Journey to Health: A Holistic Approach to Ehlers-Danlos Syndrome* by Mysti Reutlinger. Here our family found even more hope! We could get in control of our lifestyle and see better days ahead. It was then I realized our family was on a journey and we could face this head on with inspiration!

Our family has since changed our lifestyle to a more holistic approach and has enabled us to get on top of EDS and our treatment! I have a new outlook on Ehlers-Danlos Syndrome and have been inspired to help my family and others with this connective tissue disorder find hope within themselves on this journey. From those first stepping into this new world to those simply feeling defeated, I would say, "You are not alone! You are your biggest advocate. Never give up. You might have a genetic connective tissue disorder and some of the comorbid conditions are downright miserable, but we can fight this because we are stronger together."

WRITTEN BY ASHTON NESMITH-KOCHERA

I am 27 years old and live in West Virginia with my family. I have a degree in teaching and have been a certified Doula for over 7 years. Unfortunately, at this time I am left disabled due to comorbid conditions of EDS. I now advocate for EDS with hopes to raise awareness and inspire others on their Zebra journeys!

Follow Ashton's journey at **PassionateZebra.com**

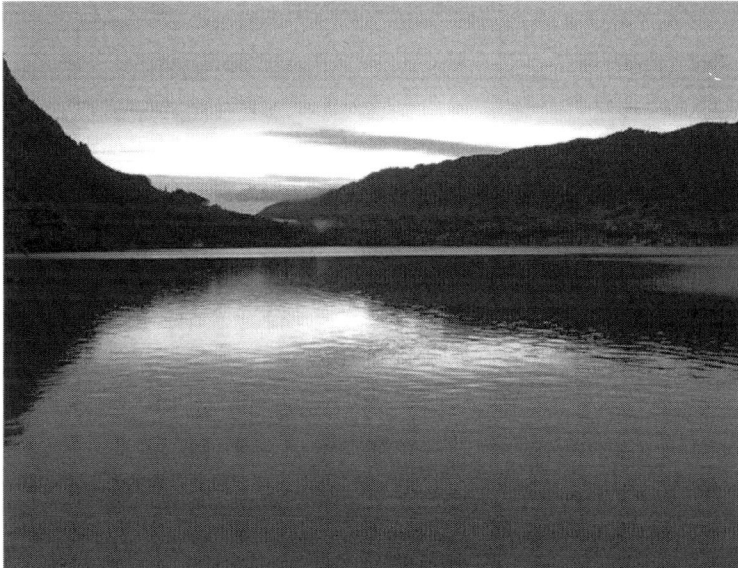

Hope is being able to see that there is light despite all of the darkness. – Desmond Tutu

Conquering EDS

I rolled over to the edge of my bed grasping at my forehead. It was day four of my migraine. As I opened my eyes and looked at the clock, I absolutely dreaded attending the occupational therapy session that I was scheduled for in one hour. I lay there contemplating what to do and decided that canceling my appointment today was absolutely necessary. Something just didn't feel right. I swung my legs around the side of the bed, hanging my head, sitting there for a while. Mornings are typically slow for me. When I finally gathered the strength to stand up, I stumbled downstairs into the kitchen to cancel my appointment. Sluggishly, I wandered up the steps stopping in the bathroom to wash my face and brush my teeth before returning back to bed to rest. Looking in the mirror was devastating. The color of my skin was so pale, my eyes were so tired, and the pain was so visible. Leaning my entire body against the sink, I turned on the water, cupped my hands and splashed it on my face. Before I knew it, things took a turn for the worse. My lungs felt like they were crumbling. There was a terrible ringing inside of my ears. I could not breathe, but surprisingly, I was extremely calm. This was the end – I was dying. I had to be. My husband, Stephen, was just around the corner sleeping in bed, but there was no voice inside of me to scream for him. Slowly, my vision began to tunnel and faded to black…

Had I gone blind!? I could not see anything, but I was still conscious. My mind was still working. I began waving my hands around across the top of the sink scrambling for a water bottle. I found it somehow by the grace of a higher being. The lid was already off. I brought the bottle to my lips and started guzzling. I instinctively backed myself over to the toilet to sit down. Slowly, my vision started to return in strange black and white pulsating patterns. So many thoughts were racing through my mind. When I felt balanced enough to gain my composure, I walked to the bedroom to wake up Stephen and explain to him what I had just experienced. He immediately noticed that I was not well, put me back into bed, handed me another bottle of water and made me something to eat. I took the current medications that I was prescribed at the time.

Next, I called a concierge doctor whose care I was under at this time. At this point I was undiagnosed. This doctor was supposed to be the best of the best. Available 24/7 for all of my needs. Recreating my experience for him, he simply stated, "Sounds like your blood pressure dropped. Stay hydrated. Let me know if it happens again." My soul was crushed. I knew in my heart this experience was so much more than that. I became infuriated, but this became the beginning. The turning point of when Stephen and I become the biggest advocates for my health.

As the months passed, my symptoms progressed. We actively searched for knowledgeable caring doctors, any type of relief, but were getting nowhere. I kept comparing what I could do today to what I could do a month ago and it was always significantly less. The end result was the purchase of a wheelchair…I was at my weakest point. My arms weren't working like they used to. I could no longer open jars, drive my car, turn doorknobs, use my fork to eat spaghetti, walk up a flight of stairs, and take a shower. Every single simple task was exhausting. My daily life was depleting.

Having faith that everything happens for a specific reason, I now realize that I had to hit my lowest point before I could set out on the journey to reach my highest. As Stephen could no longer stand to literally see me waste away, he focused ALL of his free time on searching for every possible solution to help heal me. He explored physical therapy, massage therapy, acupuncture, holistic healing, different foods, health centers, etc. During this search, I was diagnosed with classical & hypermobility EDS, POTS Syndrome, and a gamut of other medically related syndromes and diseases. I still could not find a solution on how to physically feel better. I was losing weight. The chronic pain and fatigue were wearing me down to the point where all I did was sleep and work. I was missing family functions, time with my husband, and time with my friends. I was missing out on life.

As our search for a solution continued, we discovered juicing, supplements and MOVEMENT. Yes, movement! "Just five minutes per day," states Kendra Neilsen Myles. Stephen found Kendra, one of my biggest encouragements through Instagram! An extremely busy woman herself, she gave up more of her time to inspire and educate me on the illness that we share. With her help, I was able to get out of bed and find my body again through simple things like walking, stretching, squats, calf raises, etc. Simple exercises that I can do for "Just five minutes!" Every time I'm too tired, or feel too weak, I hear those words and use my five minutes to stretch or exercise because I know that it is more beneficial for me in the long term.

With Stephen's help, I entirely changed my diet. Focusing on eating only organic foods, juicing for breakfast, replacing prepackaged foods with fruits, vegetables, and salads. Basically, only eating clean, fresh food. After about two weeks of eating clean, I even noticed that my taste buds changed! It was really hard at first. I had awful cravings for all of the junk food I was addicted to eating (cheese sticks, cheese steaks, Doritos, Fritos, Cheetos, crap, crap and more CRAP!), but I got through it! The more healthy food I ate, my cravings changed. The more movements I made, the stronger and healthier I felt.

It started with a simple walk per day, increasing little by little, only pushing myself slightly. In no time I was back in the actual gym! Stephen got me a gym membership with a prescription to the therapy pool. The therapy pool is one of my favorite ways to exercise. The warm water is beyond soothing on my joints. It allows for much easier movement. With this wonderful addition, within a few weeks, I was feeling fantastic! Better than I have felt in years! My mind even felt sharper. I was thinking so clearly!

I rolled over in bed yesterday morning thanking the universe that I am alive, that I woke up today. I am now on a new journey! I will no longer let EDS control my life. I am proud to be a Zebra and blessed to be challenged every day. With my new-found knowledge and strength I am convinced that part of my new journey is to help and encourage others as Kendra and Stephen have helped me. Each day, I remind myself to be positive and fearless. I have the ability to control all of this. With dedication, passion, gentle exercises, hydration, a few cute pairs of compression socks, and an open mind you also can live a life without regret.

Everyone is battling something. You can learn so much by listening to someone else's hoof beat. Be each other's biggest supporter, and most importantly support and love yourself.

WRITTEN BY ASHLEY PIRSCHL

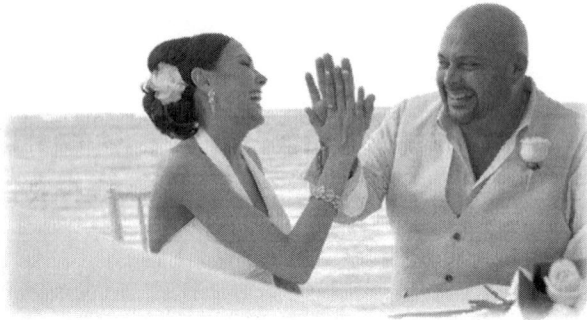

Song of the Zebra

Our hoof beats, beat along the shores of life,
we climb the pillars of pain,
and wade through sceptic seas.

For us life alters,
our hoof beats forever chase the wings of time,
but life goes on.

One day we reach dry land again,
yet we tread with caution,
wild animals hinder our return,
they hunger for us.

Our white coats gleam with sweat,
we have tried before,
many times,
but this time we'll succeed.

With our heads raised high,
we paw the ground,
and battle forward.

We'll earn our distinguished markings,
those black stripes of bravery,
that represent our own uniqueness.

We race once more,
towards our freedom.

Our hoof beats, fly along the shores of life,
we follow the invisible,
we do not fear what we cannot see,
we embrace it, determinedly.

Finally, we've been heard.
The song of the Zebra has just begun.

WRITTEN BY BECKY LOU

Becky Lou is a writer from BC, Canada. Her work has appeared in anthologies on Amazon. She is currently revising her Young Adult novel.

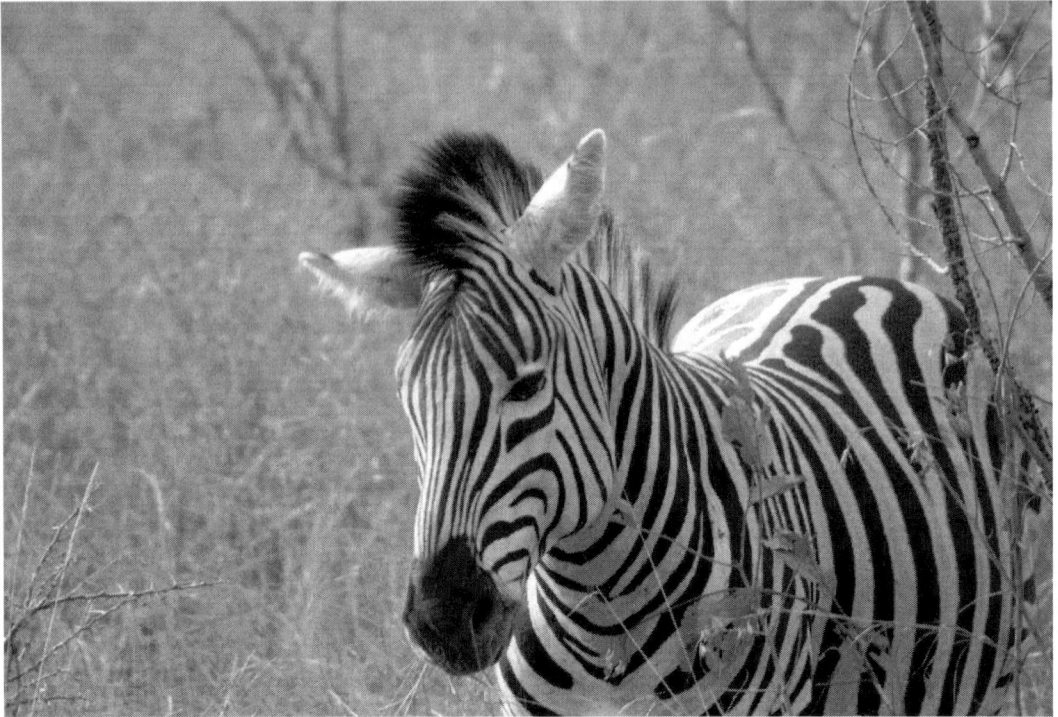

Conquering the Water

I've learned to love being in the water. Being immersed in water helps my muscles relax and allows me to move my body in ways that are far more strenuous on land.

I've spent years doing various aqua therapy programs, which have helped improve my mobility in many ways. Over time, I gained an appreciation for the water, and a new-found reverence for the immense power it held over my healing process.

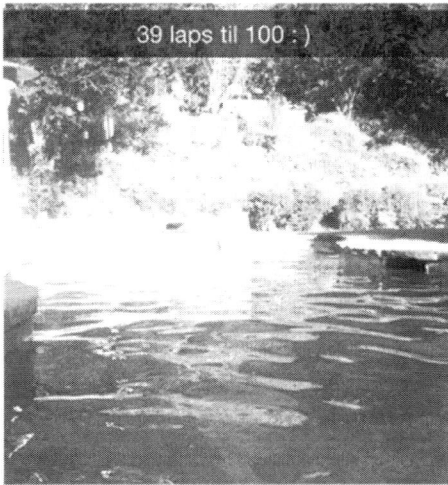
39 laps til 100 :)

One day, I was staring out at a friend's pool, admiring the way the sun reflected off the water. We had just come back from a long hike, and I decided I wanted to conquer movement in the pool in a way I never had before. With that, a new goal was formed: one hundred laps, there and back.

I knew it would be a challenge and I could not accomplish such a feat on the first try, but that was okay. I made the commitment and devoted the summer of 2013 to my hundred-lap challenge.

I hopped into the pool and mentally committed to starting with five laps, there and back. I took a deep breath and began to swim. As I completed the five laps, something inside propelled me to keep going. Five laps turned into ten, and soon enough ten turned into fifteen.

As I continued swimming, I assessed the condition of my body and pushed for just a few more laps. Exhausted, I made it to eighteen laps on my first swim of the season. What a thrill! That afternoon, I went from never swimming a lap in my life, to swimming eighteen!!

Knowing that I could conquer eighteen laps, I set a new goal of twenty-five for the next time. Again, I took to the water and swam with my whole heart. My goal came and went as I pushed myself harder. Thirty-eight, thirty-nine… forty laps! Once again, I had exceeded the goal I set for myself and it felt amazing.

My friends and family supported my goal by encouraging me to continue to push myself in healthy ways. They encouraged balanced nutrition, drinking plenty of water, and reapplying sunscreen as needed. They cheered me on throughout the process, giving me greater strength and determination to succeed with my goal.

As my journey to reach one hundred laps continued, I let go of everyone else's opinions of how I should be swimming and listened to my body's intuition as it guided me along each stroke of each lap. It didn't matter that I didn't use the "perfect form" or that I used multiple strokes to get to the end of the pool. Each lap built upon the last, and with each one I gained greater strength and stamina.

After months of practice the day arrived; I was finally going to conquer this goal. One lap after the last, in succession, I approached my goal with excitement. Ninety-eight… ninety-nine… one hundred!

What seemed to be an impossible goal not only became possible with great support and encouragement from people in my life, it was met with exhilaration that spilled over into each area of my life. I conquered the water and continue to conquer living with Ehlers-Danlos Syndrome every day.

WRITTEN BY BRIANNA GREENSPAN

Brianna Greenspan, a 27-year-old Ehlers-Danlos Syndrome (EDS) patient from California by way of Texas, is on a journey from illness to wellness. While she once lived a life defined by pain, she now lives a life driven by passion. One of Brianna's greatest passions is to help others find their own sense of strength and purpose. She believes everyone has a higher calling in life, but in order to achieve the best sense of self, one needs the necessary resources and the right support system.

Brianna strives to be a resource for the invisible illness community and currently, works as a wellness coach and consultant. She also researches EDS and the spectrum of strength and weakness within the hypermobile community alongside leading Connective Tissue Disorder specialists, Dr. Alan Weinberger, Dr. Pradeep Chopra, and Dr. Vladislav Shut. Through her social media presence and various other projects, Brianna establishes that the labels other people impose do not define a person; you can be strong if you choose to be. She has worked with over 200 patients with Ehlers-Danlos Syndrome and is in the process of creating an online EDS Wellness Coaching program to help ensure other patients have access to resources and have the tools to make it back to health. More information on this EDS Wellness program can be found at **ZebraCommunity.com**

Follow her on Instagram **@drbri1111**, or find her Facebook, **Brianna's Medical Journal**.

Nothing in this world can take the place of persistence. Talent will not; nothing is more common than unsuccessful men with talent. Genius will not; unrewarded genius is almost a proverb. Education will not; the world is full of educated derelicts. Persistence and determination alone are omnipotent.
- Calvin Coolidge

GROWTH

Without continual growth and progress, such words as improvement, achievement, and success have no meaning. – Benjamin Franklin

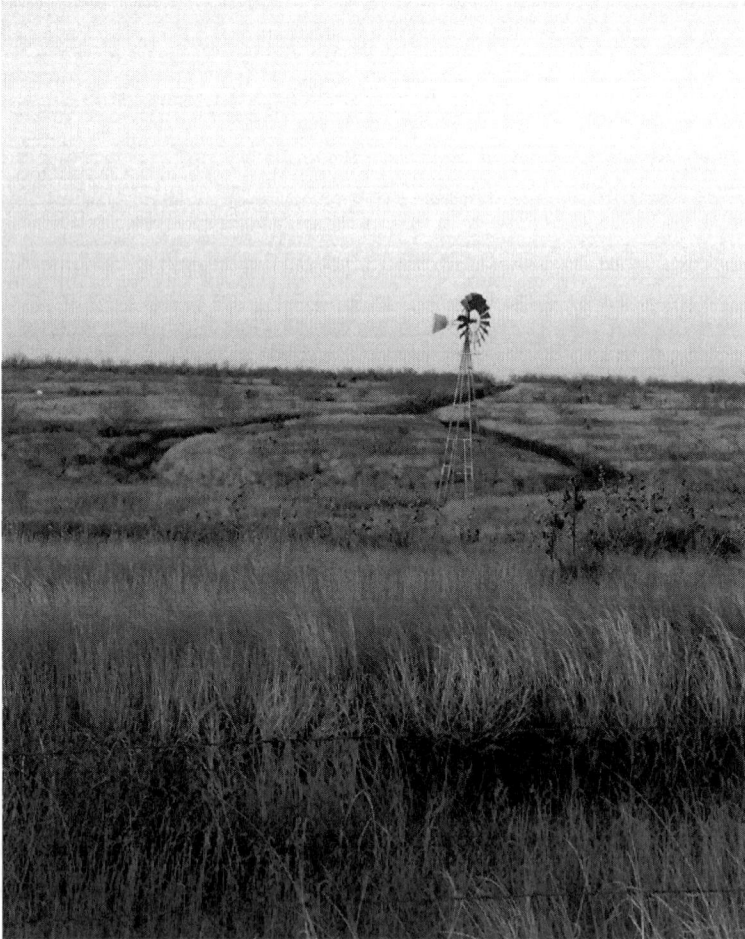

Photo by Gwynne Moore

The Worst and Best Day of My Life

I always had issues as a child, but I never noticed them. When I was little, I had something called 'growing pains' in my legs, my hips would partially dislocate or sublux, and I needed to sleep often. As I aged, I began experiencing tension headaches and severe digestion problems to the point where I could not eat without a bathroom nearby. This was incredibly annoying, but I refused to allow these problems to influence how I lived my life. I was always motivated to be the best in every endeavor.

At the age of 20, I decided to start studying for a job as a lab technician. At the time of graduation, I was elated to be ranked at the top of my class. I was awarded a wonderful position in research, moved into my first apartment, played volleyball, and had many friends. After one year of employment, I booked a trip to Italy and reveled in sunny days on the beach with friends. I had worked diligently to achieve each of these goals and life was perfect!

I only had one problem – my headaches became worse. There was excruciating pain between my shoulders and I scheduled an appointment with orthopedics. In years past, I would have massages that seemed to help my headaches. But something inside of me said that this would be different and I couldn't shake the foreboding feeling.

This time, no massage was offered or suggested. The orthopedic wanted to do injections in my neck. I reluctantly agreed. In a matter of minutes, my heart rate increased, I had numbness on the left side of my body, blurred vision, pins and needle sensations, difficulty breathing, and many more neurological issues. I had never felt such fear for my life or of anything before. Those injections nearly killed me and I found myself facing the worst day of my life.

For months, I struggled with the same symptoms. I saw specialist after specialist; each with no answers. Many doubted what I was experiencing and suggested I was depressed, burnt out, or afflicted with some other mental disorder. How could they believe this when I was living the life of my dreams?

Frustrated and with seemingly nowhere to turn, I began to research my symptoms myself in every clear moment I had (which were few). I read about the burning, clicking, cracking, dizziness, and neurological disorders. All of the symptoms continued to point to a single disease: craniocervical instability or CCI. Dumbfounded, I could not believe all the doctors I had seen were unable to see the problem!

In my research, I discovered there were only a few physicians who were able to diagnose this type of disease. I made some calls and was scheduled to see one of them. With much imaging, I was not only diagnosed with CCI, but also instability of my lower spine and osteoarthritis. My spine resembles that of an old lady! In receiving the diagnosis, I was both shocked and happy. I thought proper diagnosis would cause some doctors to believe my symptoms and work with me to help get rid of the problems.

Three years came and went. They were the hardest of my life. I traveled all around the country, did every type of physical therapy I could find, and still my disease progressed. I lost my job, my apartment, my boyfriend, many friends, and worst of all, trust in myself. More and more of my joints became unstable, my skin started to hang, and my muscles continued to lose strength; no matter how often I did muscle-building exercises. I was on my knees. Still, though the problems were increasing and my strength was fading, I had the resolve deep inside to fight this disease – even if it took my lifetime savings to do so.

I researched specialists outside of my country. In that research, I found a physician in the United States who could do therapy to stabilize the ligaments around my cervical spine. I was excited for the possibility to regain my life. I arrived in the US and began the treatment protocol. After 10 visits, my symptoms had not improved in the slightest.

Since I was already in the United States, I sought out a neurosurgeon. I figured it was worth taking a chance to see if they could help. As I was researching physicians who could handle my medical case, I came across a blog of a woman who had the same experiences as me. Nobody believed her until she saw one physician who literally saved her life. I phoned the office and they were able to squeeze me in a month later. I was terrified. I simply couldn't handle another disappointing experience.

Who would have thought that I could fly around the United States as a foreigner with very little English vocabulary and a host of medical issues by myself? That's exactly what I did as I packed my suitcase and boarded a plane because there simply was no other choice.

The day had come of my appointment. I spent three hours in the doctor's office. This doctor did not doubt me or my symptoms at any point in our conversation. He was able to piece together the puzzle that began early in childhood and diagnosed me with one primary condition:

Ehlers-Danlos Syndrome, hypermobility type.

I had heard of it before, but I was not sure what this diagnosis would mean for me now. The specialist also diagnosed me with a totally unstable cervical spine. I found out that I'd had many wrong treatments and wrong diagnoses. This was nothing I could just fix. This is a severe chronic condition that will accompany me for the rest of my life and I had to plan my life in a different way.

I learned some time after my diagnosis that this physician was not just any specialist – he is a leading expert in both EDS and CCI! Many people travel from around the world to see him for corrective surgery. It was a miracle that the office squeezed me in otherwise I'd likely still be without help.

Answers meant the beginning of a new life – my life with EDS and CCI. I made the decision to do something I did well since I could no longer work at the age of 28: I decided I would fight for myself and for all the other people in my country who have the same health problems. I built a website, a support group, wrote articles and a book. I created a YouTube channel, a Facebook page, and I found a way to connect with many EDS experts around the world. Through all of this, I've learned the value of friendships around the world and just how strong I can be by making the choice to do something that matters.

A doctor recently said to me, "There is a reason why you have this particular disease and not someone else. I believe that is because you have to build something great out of this situation." That doctor is right and I'm preparing to build an organization for patients with CCI in my country and I'm doing all that I can to raise awareness.

There will be many more fights before these rare diseases are recognized in my country. What I achieved in the hardest time of my life was so much more than I did when I was healthy. For all I lost, I gained even more. It is worth it to fight because someday everything will change for the better. I want to be the one who helped it change.

WRITTEN BY KARINA STURM

Follow Karina's journey at: **Instabile-halswirbelsaeule.de** *Edited by Mysti Reutlinger to accommodate Karina's primary language of German.*

The "I Can't" Monster

When I was nine, I was running. Then *snap* and I fell to the ground, instantly. "I broke my leg! I broke my leg!" My mother came to collect me from school. And running on the playground became something that filled me with fear.

When I was twelve I was roller skating in the car port, along with everyone on my street. Spinning and twirling. Then my leg twisted under me. I hung up my roller skates for good that day.

Before my thirteenth birthday I had knee release surgery on both knees, and I had become afraid of being active. I happily took my doctor's notes and excused myself from physical education. I avoided sports like it was something that would hurt me if I got anywhere near it.

By the time I was thirty-six, walking up the stairs had become difficult. I knew it was time to change, time to get fit, and time to become active. Intuitively I KNEW that being active would help me to feel better.

And then I dislocated my elbow. And dislocated it again. And again.

It would have been so easy to focus on the correlation between the times I tried to be active and each dislocation I had along the path. It would have been easy to surrender – to choose the fork in the road that led to "Do Nothing Ville."

But I chose the other road. The road to active living.

For almost ten years, so much of what I have done has involved pushing beyond my deep physical memories and confronting my "I CAN'T" feelings.

When I did the *Strong Like Bull* cycling training camp, Coach John Hirsch gave me the following feedback:

"…There may have been a lot of people who instead of pushing you pulled you back because of your disability… You need to be more the boss of you. You know what you can do and what you can't. You will need to keep pushing to find that edge. Once you go over it a few times you will have the experiences needed to know what you can and can't do and where that line is…"

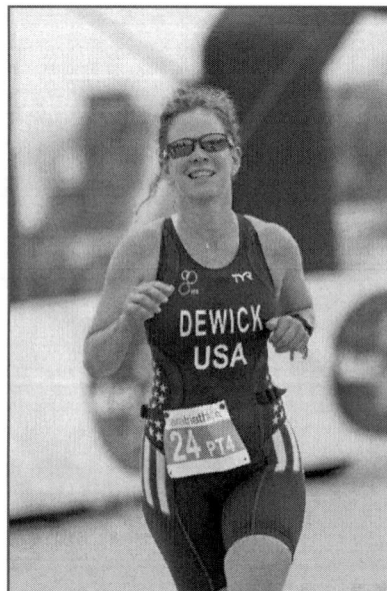

John helped me to see that I have an "I Can't Monster" living in my head.

I think my "I Can't Monster" is a monster whose heart is made up of memories of pain, whose head is full of the words from doctors who allowed me to do nothing physical, doctors who encouraged me to avoid doing things that put me at risk of pain and injury. My "I Can't Monster" is a monster with flawed collagen, whose knees are on the back of his legs, whose elbows can't support his own weight. He has a body like Gumby. He is the monster in my head that stops me from pushing myself.

Ever since my decision in 2007 to do my first triathlon, I have battled my "I Can't Monster." It is SO HARD. Each time I confront the "I Can't Monster" I push myself into unknown physical territory, into uncomfortable mental situations. I am doing things I don't ever remember doing. I am facing underlying fears. I assess the risks in each step that I take.

Each step is a victory. I am nurturing a newborn called confidence. Physical and mental confidence.

And I am the healthiest and happiest I have ever been.

WRITTEN BY DONNA DEWICK

Donna DeWick is an endurance athlete with Ehlers- Danlos Syndrome and Charcot Marie Tooth disease. She has completed numerous long distance swims, cycle rides, and triathlons since 2007, including winning a bronze medal at the International Triathlon Union World Paratriathlon Event Chicago in June 2014. She writes about her journey to active healthy living while managing chronic conditions on **BeatingLimitations.com**

Photo courtesy of Cyn Lawrence Photography.
CynLawrence.com

Bittersweet

"Oysters and Pearls" 'Sabayon' of Pearl Tapioca with Island Creek Oysters and White Sturgeon Caviar

This past winter, in an incredibly lucky turn of events, I scored a reservation for two at the French Laundry in Napa Valley. This was my mecca – the birthplace of California cuisine and Alice Water's and Thomas Keller's restaurants. The Laundry is one of the top restaurants in the world, and securing a reservation is next to impossible. I had read and heard lore about this place for the last twenty years. It was my bucket list meal. Working in the kitchen would have been my dream job. I don't think I was as excited on my wedding day as I was the night my husband and I dined there. The service was like a dance, like being a part of the most incredible performance art you could imagine. I spent half of the dinner enjoying the hell out of myself, and half of it staring enviously at the staff, wondering how they were so lucky – and how I got the short-end-of-the-stick genetically. There's no better way to describe it than bittersweet.

"Brokaw Avocado Salad" Hawaiian Hearts of Peach Palm, Compressed Cucumbers, Aji Dulce Peppers Toasted Cashews and Cilantro

I knew when I was 12 years old that I wanted to be a chef. I remember the exact moment – I was sitting outside on a hot Texas day, lost in *Gourmet* magazine. There was an article about the Culinary Institute of America (CIA), and I just KNEW that I was going to end up there. This was right before *Food Network* took off and before being a cook was a "hot" job. Everyone in my family thought I was nuts. "You're smart. Go to college. Don't waste your life in a kitchen." Yet it's where I'm most comfortable – the one place where my brain stops spinning and my body relaxes; where I know exactly what to do.

There are no insurmountable problems in a kitchen – the only goal is to make the business money, people happy, and ensure quality food at every step. It's also an incredible creative outlet. When I pick up a knife and start chopping I feel my purest self. It's the only thing I've ever found that excites every sense in my body. There is no tiredness – more satisfaction of a job well done than the exhaustion I felt after a good double-shift on the line. I was GOOD at what I did. I still understand food in a way that I don't get about life in general. I would stand up to macho ex-cons, earning my nickname of "Skinny-Strong." I was generally the only woman in the back during a shift and I held my own. I had a good feel for pastry especially – and I have one hell of a palate and a perfumer's nose. It showed.

Sweet Butter Poached Maine Lobster- Chanterelle Mushroom 'Ravioli', Sweet Garden Carrots, Cipollini Onions and Parsley

I worked hard and graduated a year early from high school, put myself through college to earn a finance degree, and then was accepted into the Baking and Pastry Certificate program at the CIA in Hyde Park, NY. I was having dizzy spells, a permanent migraine, and many other Ehlers-Danlos Syndrome symptoms common in comorbid conditions; but every doctor I saw at the time referred me to therapy or said I had too much stress, a hormone imbalance, or nothing was really wrong. I simply pushed through. What other choice did I have?

After doing well in the program and graduating, I moved to New York City to live with my fiancé and scored a position as a pastry cook at a great restaurant. I had big plans to work for a few years, earn a few promotions, and secure an amazing reputation so I could eventually open my own restaurant. Then, everything changed…

I started fainting. After hitting my head on a Hobart mixing bowl during a syncopal episode and my sous-chef believed I was faking, I went into survival mode. In this industry, you never leave a shift in the middle of service unless it is an absolute emergency. I gave notice at the restaurant and began working in an office using my finance degree. I hated it! Brain-fog was steadily creeping in and affecting my performance, but at least it was a job. My dizziness and syncope became worse and I fainted again in the car. Thankfully my husband was driving and took me to the ER. The physician ordered a tilt-table test and diagnosed me with POTS. Which meant I wasn't crazy and there really was something wrong with me.

"Wolfe Ranch White Quail" Cauliflower Cream, Preserved Meyer Lemon, Spanish Capers and Wild Arugula

My husband and I moved to Hawaii after the wedding on the advice of my headache specialist. The barometric pressure is more stable here than anywhere on the mainland. It's been seven years since we moved here and I've given birth to one child, fought for disability and won after a three-year battle. I was in poor physical shape and so improperly medicated that for over a year I would faint every time I stood up and was wheelchair-bound. My life became more isolated with numerous ER visits and hospitalizations. We had to hire a nanny help take care of our toddler. No one could figure out what was wrong with me! Doctors disagreed on what was wrong and said I had anxiety, POTS, fibromyalgia, and even conversion disorder. None of them could explain why I was so sick and why my symptoms were all over the map. I was frustrated and numb. I was consumed by not being able to follow my passions, what I was supposed to do. I was angry, barely existing. The only highlights during that time were being with my family and cooking. The kitchen made all the noise fade away and pushed the pain back – for a short time anyway.

"Soumaintrain" La Ratte Potato 'Croquette', Philo Gold Apples and Whole Grain Mustard Vinaigrette

We got back to the hotel that night after dinner and my head was buzzing. I had savored the best meal of my life, by far, and I was only beginning to wrap my brain around it. The next day, I gave myself a liter of fluids through my PICC line and walked over to the French Laundry kitchen garden. They grow the majority of the produce they use in the restaurant there. It's glorious! I stood in that garden that I had read about for years, dreamt about working in, just taking in the sight. Bees were buzzing around and chickens were clucking. Tomatoes and squash stood out technicolor bright. The air smelled of compost and chlorophyll and sunshine. As I stood there, I finally broke down.

I sobbed my heart out. It was so beautiful and perfect. And I was suffering in pain, physically and emotionally. I was flooded with thoughts of doctors, well-meaning but cruel neighbors, family who didn't understand, my failed projects, the disappointments, and the agony of being a sick person trying to be a parent, spouse, and to fight each day just to get out of bed every morning without giving up forever or over medicating. It hit me all at once – the unfairness of it all. I was there, in the place I felt I was supposed to be, where I worked my whole life to be, but I couldn't be a real part of that world. I would never be a chef. That tiny spark of hope burnt out.

It was such a relief. I knew I could either look back feeling shame, hurt, envy, and anger or accept that it just wasn't going to happen for me. I had to accept that I would never be in that place the way I desired, but I opened the door to finally plan my life in a new way.

It's not easy - the physical pain is overwhelming, but there is beauty where I live, soft breezes, and good people. There's a fruit stand down the road and my neighbor's garden that I can raid. I have a well-stocked kitchen and I can still make challah on Fridays. I have a husband who loves me and whom I adore. I've got an incredible child and a goofy lab that has the makings of a stellar service dog. This is a good life.

Assortment of Desserts-Fruit, Ice Cream, Chocolate and "Candies"

I'm 34. It took 32 years to get my EDS diagnosis. In the past two years I've changed my medical team and found an excellent primary care physician. I've started sorting out each individual comorbid condition, changed my meds, altered my diet, and I am getting physically stronger. I still fight depression after multiple days stuck in bed. That's inevitable, I think.

In a way, my life truly began when I received my EDS diagnosis and I was able to learn who I really was. Everything clicked and came into focus. I've had to let go of much in my life and accept help more often than I prefer – or will ever be comfortable with accepting. It has taken time to understand and accept that there is no cure. I'm not sure this will ever not suck. I'm not spiritual or religious and don't follow the "Let go and let God" thing, however, letting go of who I thought I should be to accept the life I have has made living easier.

The most horrible thing about EDS is the lack of knowledge. There is no defined path for any of us... We are all weird in our own quirky ways and there is no set treatment protocol. I do have some control of my treatments and my self-care. I am in control of my self-image. The structures society puts in place for healthy people are broken down for those of us living with EDS. We don't all get to have the dream life with marriage, children, and careers – those dreams are often stolen from us by this disease. EDS can steal your very essence – if you let it. It did for me. I'm rebuilding the dreams of my life – and that's a start to living.

When we left the restaurant that night they sent us home with a tin of shortbread cookies and a copy of the menu. The menu is beside me as I write this. I've scattered it throughout this essay as a reminder of the world I left behind, lost potential, and a memory of one of the best nights of my life – not just because of the impeccable meal or service, but because it was the meal that allowed me to move forward. My future is beautiful and full of promise.

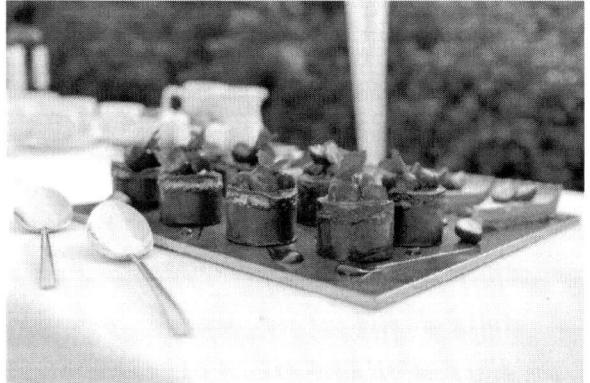

So is yours.

WRITTEN BY ALLISON WALLIS

Allison Wallis is an avid home-cook who lives with EDS, POTS, and other EDS comorbidities. She lives in Hawaii with her husband, daughter and her service dog, Pono. She loves gardening, social media, and fostering her daughter's budding feminism.

You can find her on Twitter **@AllylovesPono**

These Boots Were Made for Walking

Braces, slings, and casts. When people hear these words they cringe, but to me this is a part of my everyday life. I was born with a collagen disorder called Ehlers-Danlos Syndrome, or EDS for short. There are many different types of EDS and I have the hypermobility type that causes frequent dislocations and subluxations. It is an invisible illness and hard to detect until your body starts falling apart. Thirty percent of your body is made of collagen including muscles and organs. When mine finally really started to act up, I had no choice but to start wearing braces to stabilize my feet and wrists. I no longer had a choice; it was time to tell the truth.

I stepped out of my house, ready to brave the world. When I got to school that day, people stared and stared, I could hear whispers of awful things about me. When I tried to explain my problems for the first time everyone called me a liar and a faker. As I made my way through school that day I felt very awkward. I could not understand why no one believed me, not even my friends. After I received a ride home from school that night I cried. My mother asked me what was wrong and why I was so upset. I explained to her what had happened and she said, "There are always going to be ignorant and mean people in the world and that it was a fact of life."

One month later, my friends were getting used to me wearing braces and were starting to actually believe me after I told them to look up Hypermobility Ehlers-Danlos Syndrome and they realized I was telling the truth. My teachers soon began to realize that I was not faking it but the school nurse was very still skeptical and starting to get on my nerves. I was really getting sick of people calling me a faker and a liar. I realized that their opinions did not matter. My friends and I were so excited for the upcoming homecoming dance. They wanted to know whether I wanted to go to the dance with my big, chunky, ugly, black boots that my orthopedic specialist gave me to wear. Since I was not going to be able to dance, my friends were worried that I would not have fun, but **I** was sure I would.

The day of the dance arrived. I was so excited and I spent all day getting ready. My mother curled my long black hair with spiky blue rollers and did my make-up and nails in a sophisticated manner. I was having fun getting ready with my grandmother, aunt, sister, and mother there to watch me and share the excitement. Finally, it was time to put on my sparkly, black homecoming dress. It looked great! My mother told me that I had to get pictures with everybody. I did and it was suddenly time to go. I was excited as I walked into the dance. I was **not** going to let the fact that I could not dance get me down. Later, I realized that just because I could not dance did not mean I could not stand for small amounts of time and move my upper body to the music. **So, I did**. This caused even more conflict because I was "dancing" which meant I was faking my foot injury. I really did not care what people were saying about me because I was having fun and nothing was going to make me feel bad.

In the years following this event, I have still had people tell me that I am a faker and a liar but I do not care. I have learned that what I think of myself is more important than what others think of me.

WRITTEN BY REBECCA VANMETER

Rebecca's life since writing this story has been affected by additional symptoms and a diagnosis of fibromyalgia. She has since graduated early from high school with honors and spends her days helping her family spread awareness and supporting others. She lives with her mom, step-dad, brother, four cats and one dog. She enjoys reading (all the time), hanging out with friends, and watching Netflix.

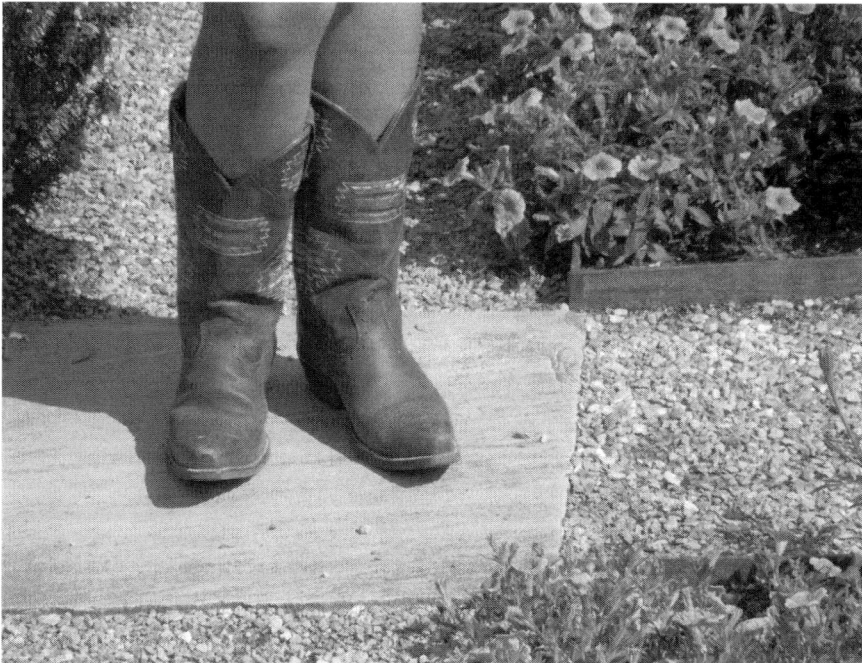

When The Pity Party's Over

I was diagnosed with Ehlers-Danlos Syndrome (EDS) at an ER at the young age of five. My mom had rushed me there, again, after what seemed like a harmless fall while roughhousing with my older sister. As the doctor stitched up the large laceration on my little leg, I watched. They questioned my bravery often, as I intently looked on as each suture was threaded. "Pretty soon you'll be a pro," the doctor joked.

I don't remember the doctor talking to my mom about my EDS diagnosis that day. All I knew was, I was five, had been to the ER more times than I could count, and knew after this I'd be able to pick out a Barbie at the toy store for being so brave. Let's just say, I had a LOT of Barbies.

What I do remember is everything that came after that day. A team of doctors and their interns would come see me once or twice a year. Asking me to do "spider fingers" with my triple jointed hands, or hooking me up to machines and talking amongst themselves while they watched the monitors. I remember the day one doctor told my mom I would need to be "exempt" from all team sports at school, and that I'd never run or even jog, and definitely not dance.

I also remember my first dance recital. I got to wear gold and black, my outfit was decidedly flashy and totally appropriate for my jazz number to "Dancin' in the Streets." It didn't hit me back then that I was 'defying' EDS. I was just a little girl living out her little dream of performing in front of a full auditorium.

My kneecap used to dislocate as often as other kids in my class sneezed. It hurt, of course, but I was pretty good at reducing it back into its place. I was a pro. I decided there was nothing physically that was going to keep me from enjoying my life. When complications from EDS struck, and they did, often, I would endure the pain, and move on. As long as I got a Barbie for my bravery.

As I got older, the realization that I was "different" became clearer. I had scars I was ashamed of. In high school, no amount of Barbie dolls made me feel more confident about my condition. My mom worried about me, of course, and her constant need to protect me made me feel like I wasn't allowed to be a teenager. And still, EDS would happen. And I would persevere, and I would move on. There's nothing those of us with EDS want more than to be labeled "normal." Even if we're not.

Fast forward to 2007. I had a fall that was more serious than any I'd previously endured. I destroyed every tendon in my knee, but worse, had severed a major artery in my leg. I underwent a total of four surgeries and months of post-surgical therapy. I had lost my job, most of my friends, and most importantly, I lost my purpose. I lived on the couch and could tell you everything on television. I was depressed and overwhelmed with thoughts of "why me?"

One sleepless night I decided to pray. I couldn't remember the last time I had. I just started talking, out loud, to God. I told Him how I didn't understand why this was happening to me, that I was angry, and just wanted to go back to being a "normal" 26 year old. My prayer went on for hours.

The next morning I felt completely different. I began journaling my experience with EDS. I began really looking at everything I'd been through, and it hit me: I am blessed beyond measure! An accident that could have taken my leg or my life, DIDN'T! I was still here, still breathing, on my way to a full recovery. And yes, life with EDS is painful, and sometimes it just plain stinks. Most who come into your life will have no idea of the struggles you endure. But you DO endure! I thought about how strong I was. The strength I realized I possessed made me feel even stronger. If I could do all this, what couldn't I do? I was no longer afraid of my life with EDS, I was empowered. Family and friends used to lament how 'strong' I was often, but I didn't believe them – and I finally saw myself through their eyes. I am an EDS Warrior!

This was not the last battle I faced. In fact, I've faced a lot since then. I can't lie and say that each time it doesn't hurt, physically and emotionally. I can't say I haven't shed many tears and asked "why me?" and thrown myself the most fabulous pity parties. I have. But now, something different happens – After the tears dry and the (pity) party's over, I remember: I can do this. There's NOTHING I can't do.

I have Ehlers-Danlos Syndrome. But it does NOT have me.

WRITTEN BY BLAIR DRISCOLL

Southwest Florida native, fashion and lifestyle blogger, medical practice manager, passionate EDS Awareness advocate.

Learn more about Blair at **BlairDriscoll.com**

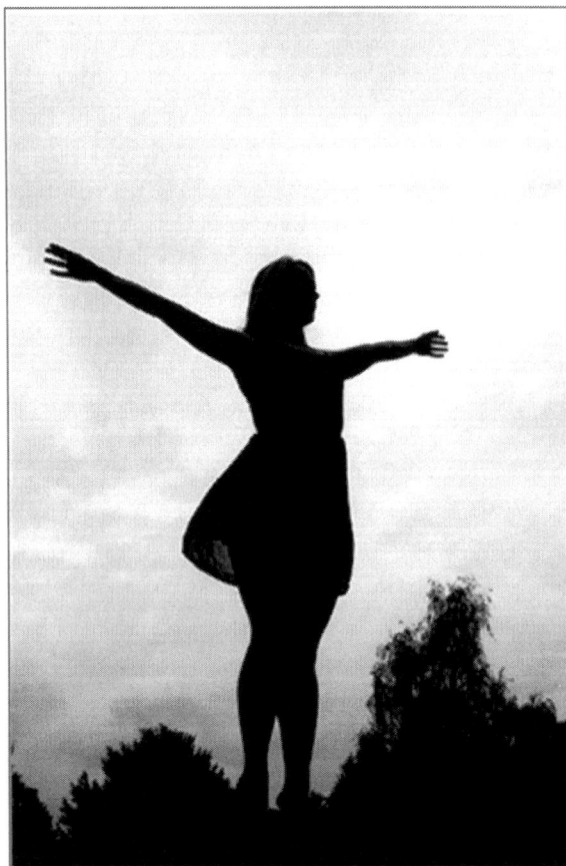

The strength I realized I possessed made me feel even stronger. If I could do all this, what couldn't I do? I was no longer afraid of my life with EDS, I was empowered. -Blair Driscoll

Living on Earth

A Survival Guide for Martians

"Why does seemingly minor trauma induce severe sometimes life-changing symptoms?" – Clair Francomano MD, Ehlers-Danlos National Foundation Learning Conference, 2011

- First, accept that you are an alien, so what's good for Earthlings may not be good for you.
- Pay close attention to your body to learn which activities hurt you. Your body may only whisper, so listen up.
- Believe your body even if your doctor doesn't.
- Become an amateur occupational therapist. You may have to modify everything you do to keep from hurting yourself.
- Eliminate or seek help with anything you can't successfully adapt.
- If no help is currently available, keep your Martian antennae out for the possibility. You never know when or from where it may come.
- If someone is interested, it's okay to tell him or her you are struggling.
- It's not okay to whine on and on.
- Never pass up an opportunity to express gratitude to those who help you and to reciprocate in any way you can.
- Smile and be cheerful as much as possible.
- Accept that sometimes things just suck, and "inspirational" messages are sent by the evil, fallen angel Satan, to torment you.
- Take responsibility for directing your own medical care. Your doctor will not know how (unless your spaceship touched down in Baltimore where there are several EDS experts.)
- Do your research. Knowledge is power.
- Don't show off your knowledge to doctors. Treat them with respect even if you think they are idiots.
- Be courteous to their staff too. Gatekeepers have power.
- Most Earthling doctors are superstitious and have been brainwashed by a misguided cult to believe that depression causes pain the way flies cause garbage. Unless you think antidepressants will solve all your problems, be cautious about the feelings you share with your doctor.
- Seek out a primary care doctor who believes your symptoms are real and wants to help. Thank and encourage her often, as she is a sensitive and endangered species.
- Martians need plenty of restorative sleep to heal the constant trauma of life on a hostile planet. It won't happen if you are in pain, or too hot, cold, stressed, or cramped. Get a good mattress that is roomy and the most comfortable bedding you can find. Relax before bed with a hot Epsom salt bath. Dim lighting, breathing exercises, and meditation are good too. Avoid

talking about or watching anything agitating on TV before bed. Take medication if you have to. You might have apnea and not know it. Try using nasal strips and avoiding sleeping on your back. Martians suffer through menopause too. If hot flashes keep you up, try evening primrose oil.

- Keep moving. If you can't make it around the block, walk to the corner. Do it again later. And then again. If you can't walk, swim. If you can't swim normally, you can adapt by using floats and reducing your range of motion to protect your shoulders. Find a pool with a handicapped lift if you need one. Warm water physical therapy relieves delicate joints from the stress of gravity and works best for many. Watch the resistance, though; you can still hurt yourself in the water. If all else fails, ask a physical therapist to show you some gentle exercises you can do in bed.

- Planet Earth gets cold. Keep your delicate body warm to break the vicious cycle of muscle tension, sleeplessness, and pain. Turn up the heat, soak in a hot tub, use a heat lamp, take a sauna, or sunbathe in the hot sand. Ice packs may not be good for you.

- Drive a minivan. The seats are higher and more ergonomic, and the ride is less bouncy than many vehicles. You can also put a bed in the back and lie down while someone else drives you. Driving a minivan also helps a Martian pass undetected in human society.

- The strain of holding yourself together under Earth's gravitational field has probably left your entire body clenched and sore. Massage may help but can be risky. Compose a short speech of do's and don'ts for the therapist to minimize the chance of injury. Look for a good student massage program in your area so that you can afford to go regularly.

- Try a topical anti-inflammatory such as Voltaren. You might be surprised by the results of putting the medication directly on the pain site rather than taking it orally.

- If your physical therapist says, "You need to push through the pain" or brings out stretchy rubber bands, deploy your antennae and vanish as fast as you can.

- If you can, go away overnight to a nice place with a hot tub. Freeing yourself from the stresses and demands of daily life will reduce your pain, renew your courage, and make you feel like a whole new Martian.

- Your species did not evolve on this planet, so some of its foods may not agree with you. Pay attention to how your body feels after you eat and adjust your diet accordingly.

- Electricity builds up in your pain sites. Ground yourself by walking barefoot on the grass or the beach. Since you are marooned on the blue planet anyway, treat yourself to a refreshing dip in its spectacular oceans. You might even feel almost human.

WRITTEN BY THE MUSE OF COMEDY

Following a seventeen-year career as a certified public accountant, the Muse of Comedy is currently cultivating her true nature as a creative. She enjoys photography, graphic arts, and origami. She lives in California with her husband and dog. She has joint hypermobility EDS.

Follow the Muse of Comedy on her blog: **StretchyGenes.wordpress.com**

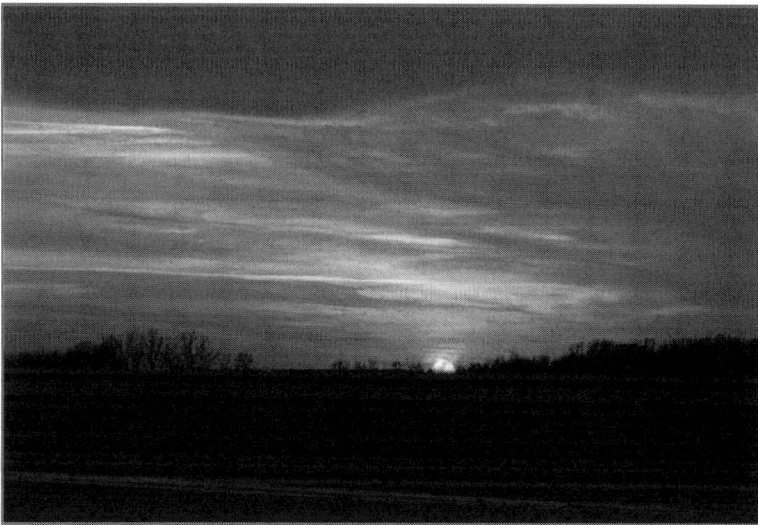

I love people who make me laugh. I honestly think it's the thing I like most, to laugh. It cures a multitude of ills. It's probably the most important thing in a person.
– Audrey Hepburn

The Hypochondriac

"Clearly there's something psychological going on here." She said this rather flatly, though the weight of it hit me like a smack to the back of the head. I stood there, in front of her, with my pants bunched gracelessly around my ankles and my mouth hanging open.

I'd requested an appointment to discuss the numerous bruises on my legs, not for a mental evaluation. Granted I probably made more appointments than the typical patient, I was—unknowingly—hot on the trail towards being diagnosed with Ehlers-Danlos Syndrome. I may not have been able to connect the dots, but I knew enough to recognize that the symptoms I was experiencing were troubling enough to seek the advice of a doctor. So why was my would-be savior writing me off as a psych case?

When the immediate shock of her accusation subsided, it was quickly replaced with overwhelming self-doubt. The doctor tiredly began to recite the protocol for submitting requests for referrals as she tapped away on her laptop, but I only caught about every third word she said.

I was mentally revisiting every recent appointment I'd ever had. I was already beginning to convince myself that maybe some of them had been a little frivolous. I was trying to reconcile issues that had once seemed very important, and now made me feel like a hypochondriac. I was also having trouble pulling my pants back up.

"Any other…" the doctor paused long enough to cross her arms and look me up and down, "…issues?"

She sat behind her computer screen, annoyance radiating from her relentless, frosty stare. I could see only from her nose, which she looked down as she waited for my response. I felt dismissed. I felt bullied and anxious as I stood there trying to swallow the lump in my throat. Why wouldn't she help me?!

Then I realized that I terrified this woman.

This woman, who had barricaded herself behind her laptop and wire-rimmed frames and cool condescension, who wrapped herself in a white coat and called herself a doctor, was nothing more than that; just a woman.

She was a woman who, like the rest of us, craved validation. However, her motivation to help me rested in the confirmation of her skills as a healer. The only problem was that she knew I couldn't be healed. I wouldn't be an easy fix or a quick boost to her ego. I might even make her question her abilities as a doctor, and that scared the hell out of her.

She no longer saw me as a patient, but a thorn in her side. I was denying her the opportunity to prove how worthy of the title "Doctor" she really was. I was a reminder that she did not have all of the answers, and probably never would.

I knew that I would not be receiving any more help from this woman, so I thanked her for her time and left her office with a referral to see a therapist. I even made the appointment and spent several lovely hours discussing every aspect of myself with a professional. We both came to the same conclusion; my issues were physical, not mental.

Since then, I have decided to act as my own advocate. I needed some serious support and no one was just going to give it to me; I had to help myself. I began scouring the Internet for information and advice. I researched specialists and read patient reviews until I knew every practitioner in the state by name. I kept diaries of my varied symptoms and brought them to my appointments. I insisted that tests were ordered and referrals sent and that I had my own copy of everything to keep track of it all. To be perfectly honest, I was obnoxious.

The countless hours I spent researching and preparing has truly served to benefit me and my relationships with my healthcare providers. I now choose to work only with doctors who are willing to work as hard as I am.

It took several years, hundreds of appointments and a lot of determination, but I was finally diagnosed correctly and began receiving the appropriate treatment.

Of course, I still run into the occasional unsympathetic practitioner. Even my own mother still asks things like, "Can't you just stop eating wheat?" But now I realize that I do not have to settle for second-rate treatment or "waste-basket diagnoses." I am not "crazy" for trying to address concerns about my health and improve my quality of life. I am not lazy for listening to my body and respecting its limitations. And, I do not allow doctors to intimidate me because, after all; they're just people.

When the immediate shock of her accusation subsided, it was quickly replaced with overwhelming self-doubt. -
Taylor Greigh

WRITTEN BY TAYLOR GREIGH

Born and raised in New Hampshire, Taylor now happily resides in Austin, TX. Taylor is a former preschool teacher, who has retired early due to complications involving her EDS. She now spends her time upcycling old furniture, playing with her dog, Scooter, and – of course – writing.

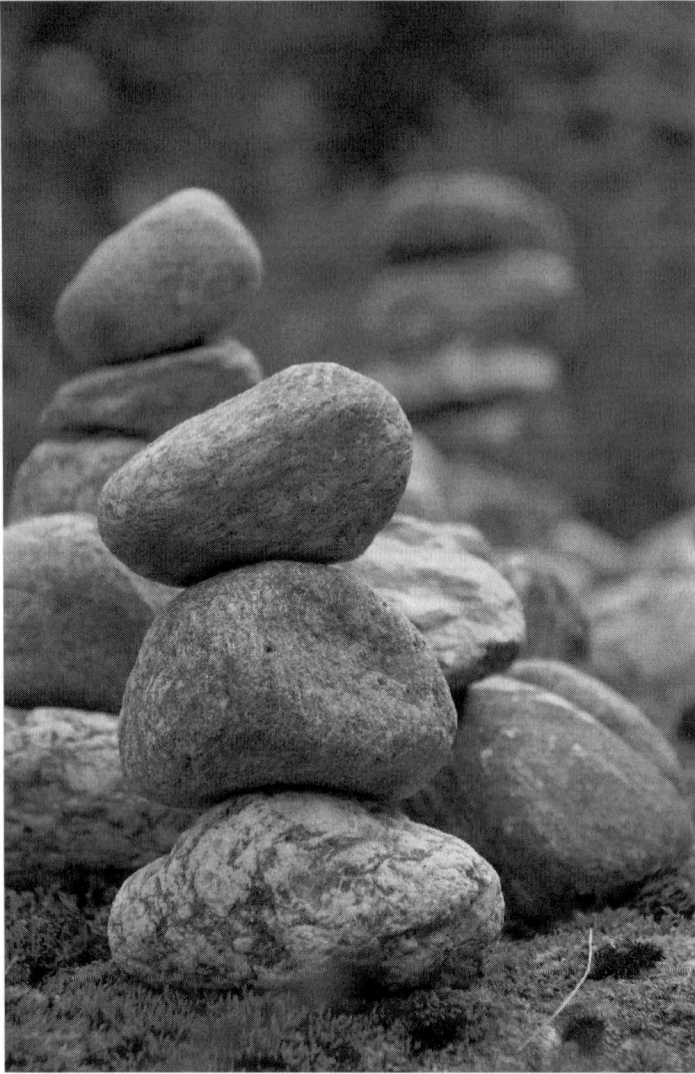

Balance, peace, and joy are the fruit of a successful life. It starts with recognizing your talents and finding ways to serve others using them.
-- Thomas Kinkade

FAITH

If patience is worth anything, it must endure to the end of time. And a living faith will last in the midst of the blackest storm. – Mahatma Gandhi

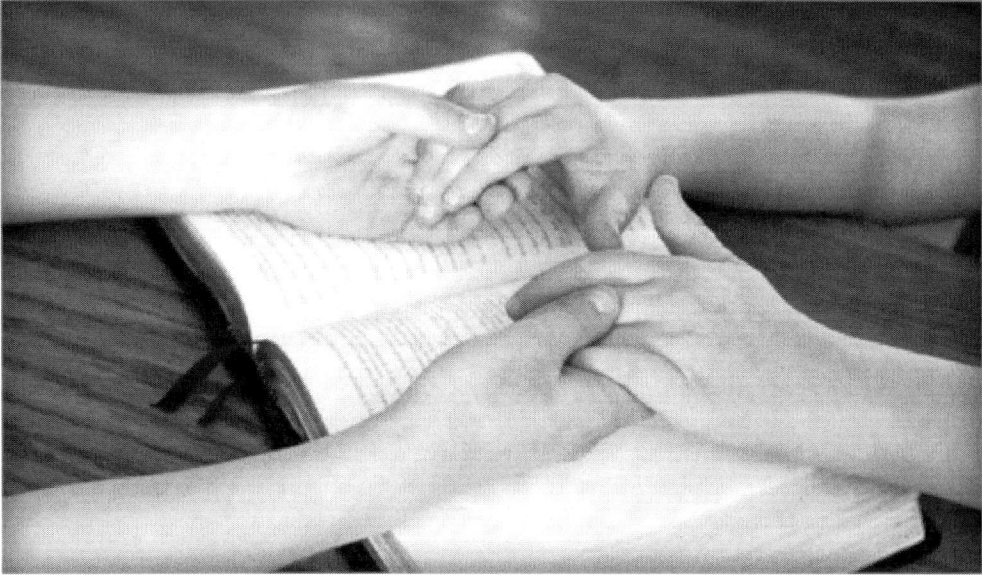

From Pity Party to Passionate Purpose

Back in the summer of 2013, I was feeling pretty defeated. After battling chronic pain for over two years, I had finally surpassed some obstacles of our local healthcare system and had been able to see not just one, but two geneticists.

I travelled out of province, to Calgary, ten hours away for my first appointment. Ironically two weeks later, I was offered an appointment five hours away in Saskatoon after waiting almost two years. Both doctors confirmed what I had suspected throughout the course of my journey to seek answers. I was now a Zebra. I guess I had always been a Zebra but I was finally going to get acquainted with my stripes at the age of 39.

I was feeling pretty sorry for myself. Besides dealing with health concerns, I had given up a short but promising career in a law firm, due to the fact that typing at a desk all day long had contributed to the onset of my pain, beginning my search for answers.

In 2011, I made the decision to return to work in my former capacity, as a home daycare provider. Being around happy youngsters seemed like it should be a pretty good remedy for my low spirits. Physically and mentally I was tired. I did however, take the entire summer off from daycare to try and relax and to recoup some of my health; emotional and physical. My spiritual life was, at this point, almost non-existent.

One evening, while in Regina to drop off my son at a high school football camp, my family and I stopped in at a popular bookstore in the city. I confess, I am a book nerd. I can spend hours browsing the displays and choosing books to bring home to my massive collection. I have shelves upon shelves in my basement; a testament to this very fact. I was an addict. I was trying to cut back. I have hundreds of books at home that haven't even been read yet!

On this particular trip, I was going to limit myself to just one book, so I had to make my choice very carefully! Little did I know, the book I selected would change my life for the better, in more ways than one!

I began to search the notes in my smartphone. Whenever a friend or family member raved about a book, if I thought I would enjoy it, I made sure to note it in my phone. I figured I had better consult my list of authors and books waiting patiently for me to read them! It was at this moment that I recalled two friends had recommended an inspirational series by a local author.

I prefer reading the work of local authors. I am a huge fan of authors from my city, province, and even just Canada in general. Canada may not be known for their high quality television production but this country is home to some of the most talented writers I have ever had the pleasure of reading! I knew I would be able to find the title I was looking for in the Regina bookstore as this unread author was based out of Lumsden, just a short drive away.

I easily found the four books in the series and picked up the first one. *Pewter Angels*, by Henry K. Ripplinger, at first glance of its shiny cover, was a very professional looking novel, featuring two angels flying about a starry sky. I had found the book I wanted to buy and I had only been in the store for ten minutes! As tempting as it was, I held back and purchased only the first book. The other three would have to wait.

We were on vacation the following week. After dropping our son off at camp, my husband and younger son and I were off to visit friends at their Turtle Mountain cabin. While my husband drove, I read. I am a lousy travelling companion, not one to make conversation while reading. I immediately was sucked into the story and characters!

A few hours later, we arrived at the cabin and I excitedly went on and on about this book to my friend. She laughed as she came out of her bedroom with a book in her hand, and asked, "Is this the one?"

She explained she had just picked it up the other day when the author was signing books in Regina! Immediately, I was jealous over the fact she had met the author! She hadn't started reading her copy yet, but based on my account of the novel so far, she planned to get into it right away!

Our visit was short but so much fun! The time spent with her family; boating on the lake, soaking up the warm sun, swimming in the cool blue water, and later, relaxing around a fire was therapy all of its own. When we said our goodbyes and my husband hit the highway, I got back into the story, forgetting about my own problems, absorbing so many life lessons found within the pages of the book. I knew that when we were back in the Regina area to pick up our son, we would be returning to the bookstore for me to grab the next three books in *The Angelic Letters Series*!

I spent the next couple of weeks lounging on the swing outside my little cottage, lying on the beach and pedaling in my paddle boat on the lake, reading page after page, torn between rushing and knowing that if I did, the books would soon come to an end. Sadly, the fifth book wasn't available in stores until the following spring!

I was hooked on the content but the perfectionist within me was disappointed with the amount of errors throughout the pages. As each book progressed, the number of mistakes grew increasingly more frequent, distracting me from the story itself. For such a professional looking publication, I felt sorry for the author. My friend and I texted each other back and forth for the rest of the summer, discussing in great detail, every aspect of the entire series. It was fun to see someone as excited over a book as I was!

I felt frustrated when book four reached its cliffhanger conclusion, but I was inspired by the characters, the choices that they made, and their decisions to seek God in troublesome situations! I was feeling so much more alive than I had in quite some time! The book spoke to my heart unlike any other book has!

I knew I had to contact Mr. Ripplinger and thank him for writing such an amazing series of books! I wanted to tell him how much they helped me conquer the pity party that had been forming inside of me. In an email at the end of the summer, I explained to him how I had just discovered the series, much too late for my liking since my friends had been talking about the books for the last two years! If only I had discovered them sooner! I politely mentioned that in my humble opinion, the proofreading needed some attention.

Imagine my surprise when Henry phoned me the next day from his residence in Lumsden just three hours away from Estevan where I live! We chatted about the books and he asked me if I would be interested in helping him out with future proofreading.

Would I? I have been blessed with an uncanny ability to uncover grammatical and punctuation problems in any material I come across on a daily basis. This was a dream come true for me!

The fourth book was going for a second printing in a just a few weeks. He wanted me to reread the book and submit to him any errors I could detect. With my copy of the book in one hand, and a highlighter in another, I set out to do the job as time was of the essence! There were many late nights just to reread the material and many more to type out any errors I could find. I was ruthless. No comma or lack thereof went unnoticed!

Poor Henry was shocked! He hadn't fathomed that there were so many corrections needing to be made. He explained that each correction ended up costing him money since the book was already set at the printers. Out of the hundreds I submitted, he chose the most noticeable 80 to be sent in for correcting. He asked me if I was interested in helping him when the fifth book in the series went to print.

We kept in touch and a few months later, I received the manuscript for the fifth book, *Angel Promises Fulfilled*. I was on cloud nine! I was getting a sneak peek into the author's mind, his world, his characters, and his story! I was in the comfort of my home and I was working so to speak, doing something I enjoyed more than any other job I had ever been employed to do. I was also being compensated for my time!

This fall, *Pewter* Angels was released in the United States. I was consulted to help compile a list of questions for a study guide at the back of this book. It was a joy to reread the book that helped me get my life back on track again!

There is one more book in the series to be written. I look forward to the day when I can be of service again. Since working with Henry, I have made another contact in the publishing world and hope to work for her some day in the future. While I am still doing daycare, my own children are almost grown and I am hoping to branch out into something new, despite the challenges EDS has cluttered in my path. I am feeling much more confident than I was a few years ago.

Even though my life has not turned out the way I might have planned, I am no longer feeling sorry for myself. God has a plan. I have a new-found purpose. Helping such a well-known author has been an honor for me. Writing has been a lifelong dream of mine. I see the work that I am doing today could potentially be a stepping-stone to fulfilling that dream.

Like the characters in the books I have become a fan of, I have grown. I am feeling more content with what I have and do not focus on what I have lost. I have a renewed faith in God my Father. I am happy to serve others as I truly believe that is what we are put on earth to do. What we do for a living isn't the important thing; it's how we go about doing it. I even returned to my roots this past summer and went to work at a grocery store at the little summer resort store near my cottage. I had a similar job as a teenager. It wasn't a prestigious or well-paying job but it was something I do well and enjoy!

The store owner reminded me of one of the main characters in Henry's books! I was happy to be doing something useful over the summer on my time off from daycare. I was thankful that I had found another little job that that didn't cause my body a lot of pain. I hope to return again next summer. I find that keeping busy is key to keeping my spirits up.

In Proverbs 17:22 it says: *A joyful heart is good medicine, but a broken spirit dries up the bones.* I plan to remember this for as long as I am here on this earth, no matter how I can be a service to others, no matter where the journey of life takes me, Zebra stripes and all!

WRITTEN BY JENNIFER HOWIE

Jen has been married for 20 years and is a mother to two teenage boys. She has been writing since she could hold a pen. She currently lives in the oil patch of southeast Saskatchewan but longs to head west. She currently works in an employment office and was surprised to discover her boss is a Zebra too! She keeps busy helping plan the Estevan Christian Women's After Five supper meetings.

Even though my life has not turned out the way I might have planned, I am no longer feeling sorry for myself.
-Jennifer Howie

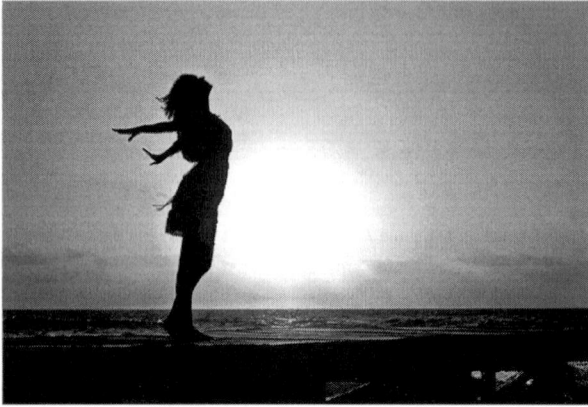

How Humor and EDS Gave Me

What I Never Knew I Needed

Before I was chronically ill, I struggled with many symptoms related to my underlying health issues my entire life. I had no idea the problems were from a condition, or a disease I simply I felt embarrassed about, or ashamed to admit it because I was surrounded by people, some of whom were friends and family, who did not understand how I could do so much, but feel awful at the same time.

To many normies, an illness means you should be incapacitated. I was often told there was no way it was that bad since I still participated in so many activities, could walk, or I didn't 'look' like I was sick. I'm not going to lie, for several years I believed them and worked harder to push past pain and symptoms making it even harder to cover up how difficult things were for me.

Now that my conditions have progressed and rendered me disabled, I shake my head at what I dealt with physically. I am glad that I have left those naysayers behind and found good, funny, and understanding friends. I have not been doubted once. Dealing with the pain and unpredictability of my conditions requires the people in my life to be flexible and understanding. To keep that, it requires me to be honest about my health with them. Not that I'm a Debbie Downer about all that goes on, just brutally and humorously honest. As I became more practiced in being truthful and appreciative of the support, I gained such indescribable liberation.

Such liberty came at high price and a challenging road. It all began New Year's Day 2005, around 3 am. My roomie and I were walking across campus after a successful and safe New Year's Eve party at a college fraternity. Poor lighting and construction caused me to pronate my foot on the curb way past the norm. X-rays determined that I had a grade-3 high ankle and lateral sprain and I had torn the tissue that keeps the tibia and fibula in place. I needed surgery, but, lacked insurance.

Three months later, I was diagnosed with Complex Regional Pain Syndrome (CRPS). Medications, physical therapy, immense pain, and coming to terms with the whole "I may never walk again" was the prescription. After a year, several cortisone shots, and doing every single exercise my PT told me to do I miraculously achieved remission. Over the next several years, I manage to stay away from a full-blown relapse, which is impressive considering I'm a major klutz and I started Irish dancing competitively. Yep, I'm pretty crazy!

Fast forward to two years ago. I was in the best shape of my life. I had a steady job, hobbies (Irish dance and service dog training), and I was finally figuring out what I could do with my passion for teaching, fitness, and dance. Then, I came down with mono January 2013. After a nearly two-week absence, I returned to work, but I never returned back to normal. My mental fatigue was awful, my muscles would fatigue more quickly when I danced. Strains and minor injuries came and went at an alarming rate. It was impossible to feel rested and to not crash after working out or dancing. I pushed through it – I even competed and placed well in competitions despite feeling as if my body was working against me.

Then one fateful day in October 2013, I was dancing in my kitchen and sprained my left ankle and strained some tendons. CRPS came roaring back. Thanks to deep denial, I continued to work despite being a gimp who couldn't stop being sick. Once again I hid my pain and struggles. December brought another illness, tachycardia, and an odd tremor that would occur randomly. Little did we know, that was just the beginning…

I was fired in January 2014 due to my failing health. Challenges continued and progressed. I started to have near-fainting spells left and right. The tremors graduated into intense shaking and twisting that spread to half of my body. I made repeat visits to the ER to receive IV medication to 'unlock' muscles that went rigid. I started to see a neurologist, and after much head scratching and tests, it was decided I had dystonia. The months dragged on and I kept getting worse.

I experienced at least 2-3 episodes of shaking, tremors, and/or twisting involving at least half my body per day. My car was sold back to the dealership, since I could no longer drive. In April 2014, my right hand clenched into a fist and has remained useless ever since. Out of nowhere, my list of food allergies grew and some reactions were so violent I should have gone to the hospital. Then my stomach/GI tract began to act up and I began to have red patches and hives after being exposed to various benign triggers. I was forced to use a wheelchair to avoid falls and my symptoms continued to worsen.

I was not completely defeated by the lack of answers. I knew there had to be someone with similar experiences. Through an amazing series of fortunate connections, I befriended an incredible young woman with CRPS on Instagram. She has an extremely adorable and great service dog named Alice Eloise. We had several things in common and we became friends. I noticed she was part of a CRPS group called CRPS PIP Support. I figured what the heck, if she likes it, it must be a good group! Through that group I received many lovely welcomes, helpful advice, understanding, and unyielding support.

In July, I landed in the hospital for five days unable to move my legs. At first the doctors were baffled, but tried tirelessly to help. Then one old navy doctor, with specialties in debunking theories of medicine, decided I was crazy. My care went from steady to non-existent as I was thrown in the 10th circle of Dante's easy bake oven. This was my lowest point. Mercifully, however, it led to the incomparable Nancy Cotterman of CRPS PIP offering to email a specialist to see if I could get an appointment. She insisted I go and CRPS PIP would help cover the expense of seeing the doctor. Miraculously, he responded to Nancy's email saying we can call his scheduling person to line up an appointment.

In September, I saw Dr. Pradeep Chopra. I was BEYOND nervous! I had heard nothing, but, great things about him. Yet still, you learn not to get your hopes up when you're chronically ill. After the exhaustive exam, intake of medical history, and showing our videos and pictures, Dr. Chopra came to his conclusions. As he began listing off my various diseases, Jon and I sat in amazement. Talk about way more information than we ever thought we'd receive on that trip!

Dr. Chopra explained that I have central sensitized CRPS, which makes treatment challenging. I am a bit of an atypical CRPS patient with secondary dystonia in multiple places from more than one disease. More diagnoses came and I was woefully unprepared for the revelations that came with it. I found out my normal in terms of pain, fatigue, and so on was all due to this… I was born with an inherited genetic connective tissue condition called Ehlers-Danlos Syndrome (EDS) and for nearly 30 years I had no clue.

Having EDS means my body and system are at risk for developing a plethora of issues. One of them is mast cell activation syndrome (MCAS/MCAD) – the nasty culprit behind my strange food allergies, severe seasonal allergies, rashes, hives, bizarre red splotches, and likely contributes to my crazy case of dystonia. He discovered that I have craniocervical instability, TMJ, and chronic daily headaches thanks to my squishy and thus weak connective tissues... He confirmed that I had POTS and dysautonomia explaining the tachycardia, low BP moments, near fainting etc. I also have gastroparesis – fortunately not a severe case. It is, however, behind many of my stomach problems. I still get nasty flares making even a small bite of food agonizing to consume. To round it off I was diagnosed with neurogenic bladder and non-restorative sleep because – why not?!

I've always said, "Go big or go home!" Just never thought it would apply to my health!

Since receiving those diagnoses, I've done a lot of looking at my past. My life has always been painful… and I mean it in the most literal sense. I have known pain since I can remember. Extreme fatigue, problems with healing, allergy issues, chronic headaches, and on and on accompanied me. My parents believed in being tough and to push through pain. In time, I figured it was better to refrain from griping as much as possible and learned to push.

My life past and present, and my pain was explained in four-ish hours with Dr. Chopra. He answered more questions than I thought I had and gave us a treatment plan to get started on. Suddenly everything was clear and my pain and struggles were validated. I was so overwhelmed that I forgot to give Dr. Chopra the biggest hug on the planet. No worries, he forgave me! I owe him and CRPS PIP everything.

It's been a crazy ride, but I do like a challenge! Overly optimistic alert! Feel free to roll your eyes when you read this: **Life is really amazing!** Don't get me wrong, though, I definitely have my days when my body isn't working, the pain is tremendous, or I just need a good cry. My life has changed dramatically! Despite being so sick, I still have a multitude of reasons to seek out the joy and fun every day. I have learned to not hide from the world. It's true, I am disabled, but that doesn't mean I've lost my value. I no longer carry my burden in secret. Living openly and honestly has brought me more inner peace than I could have ever imagined.

I have found the most supportive friends and family, service dog, and fiancé. I have learned that who you surround yourself with is crucial. They lament with me on the bad days and laugh with me at the funny and crazy moments of life. I honestly believe without them, I would have gone quite mad by now.

I can't imagine ever going back into hiding. There is too much beauty to allow me to slip into the shadows and be blinded by it. People often think that the light and dark are opposites, but, they're not. Darkness is only the absence of light; the tiny spark from a match or a candle can drive back and illuminate the darkest night. Laughter, friends, and puppy are the best medicines for me and I don't want to ever lose them. Being ill has taught me the importance of that and the importance of reaching out, sharing, and helping others. It's also the best way to stay out of my old dark corners.

I'd love to say to every person who is struggling to find their inner joy, despite their body being beaten down by disease, to keep at it. It is there! Surround yourself with people who are willing to lighten your burden in the good times and the bad. Make sure you let them know how special they are and how much they mean to you, and they will do the same. Cry when you need to, but find a way to laugh.

Be patient with yourself, it doesn't fall into place all at once. Have faith! There ARE individuals and groups out there that understand. Open your eyes a little, take a deep breath and find the right people to light up your life.

WRITTEN BY MEGAN BANNING

Megan Banning lives in Tulsa, Oklahoma with her fiancé Jon and small urban zoo of rescued cats and dogs. While currently sidelined from competitive Irish dancing and other hobbies due to her disabilities, Megan still enjoys blogging, photography, teaching piano, hanging out with friends when she can, talking to groups about disabilities and service dogs, and working with her own service dog Lady. She looks forward to more stability with her health. In the meantime, however, she won't let bad days stand in the way of loving, making the most of, and laughing at life.

Follow her blog at: **TheLifeAdorkable.com**

*It's true, I am disabled, but that doesn't mean I've lost
my value. I no longer carry my burden in secret.
-Megan Banning*

A Spiritual Journey of Healing

My story began like many others': my mother and I spent a few confusing years wondering why my health was failing at such an early age. At the age of 13, I was finally diagnosed with EDS Type III, and later with fibromyalgia. At the time, I was a star swimmer and I even became co-captain of the high school swim team. Once I attended college, however, my illness became unbearable. I looked completely normal, but I felt anything but normal. I had no other choice but to take a medical withdrawal from college. My dreams of becoming an interior architect were completely crushed and I spent the next few months bedridden, depressed, and thinking that I had no future ahead of me.

At the time, medication was the only thing that was being offered for the long-term symptomatic relief of EDS. Before I knew it, I was on a cocktail of medications. I felt hopeless, yet the medication provided me with enough juice to get me through the next few years.

Using Myspace, I created the first online Ehlers-Danlos Syndrome community on social media. Connecting with others was a godsend. Finally, we were able to share our symptoms and discover correlations that were beyond the textbook. It was truly amazing to have this resource. Even though I made a few leaps forward during this time, I eventually had to walk away from the group. It dawned on me that no one there had any answers. We were all still suffering and hearing about everyone's suffering only made me feel worse. Feeling despair, I turned away from the Internet, my friends, and even my family.

If there were one quality I've always had alive in me, it would be my child-like wonder for learning. Even through my darkest days, I had a book in my hand or the Internet at my fingertips. This phase was needed as I was now embarking on a Spiritual Journey. Without any conscious intention, I began practicing mindfulness and meditation techniques. I remembered that yoga brought me some relief in the past. Not knowing if yoga was safe for someone with EDS, however, I ended my practice years ago. Eventually, I came to the conclusion that anything was worth a shot. I began a gentle, daily yoga practice until I had a major awakening. I realized that this was really helping me. I wondered, "Is anyone else talking about this?"

Again, I took to the Internet, but there was not much information about EDS and yoga. To fill this void, I began a new group on social media: the Facebook page "Yoga for Ehlers-Danlos Syndrome & Fibromyalgia." I had more questions than answers, but I felt very passionate about my vision. In the beginning stages of the site, I wrote a story about my awakening titled: "A Spiritual Journey of Healing." Not long after, I won a contest to meet my favorite, world-renowned yogi – Rainbeau Mars. Before I knew it, I had people interested in what I was doing and we all started to find some relief. To this day, I still post positive quotes, techniques for relaxation, and online yoga videos with modifications. With the knowledge gained from my personal experience I am now committed to providing a service to others in this unique field of EDS and yoga.

It has been three years since I started this Facebook page. I have since been recognized on such sites as Shape.com and Grokker.com. When feeling inspired, I share my writings and gluten free recipes on my personal page **theglutenfreeyogi.com**. What I've learned from my journey is that the most powerful healing tool of all is connecting with others in a positive ways.

I sit here now realizing how far I've come. I'm just weeks away from completing a yoga training program. This is an accomplishment I would have previously thought was impossible. With a better understanding of yoga, I've learned to integrate EDS into my spiritual practice. Rather than fighting my illness on a daily basis, I've come to face it, use it, and feel empowered by it. I now look at EDS as my gift rather than my hindrance. With a positive, creative, and happy mindset the future can look bright for those who are ready to move forward.

My message: Be an inspiration.

WRITTEN BY CHRISTINE SPENCER

Join Christine's Yoga Community on Facebook:

YogaForEhlersDanlosSyndrome

You may not always have a comfortable life and you will not always be able to solve all the world's problems at once, but don't ever underestimate the importance you can have because history has shown us that courage can be contagious and hope can take on a life of its own. – Michele Obama

Just the Beginning

I was born in 1988 with every joint from my hips down dislocated. The physicians just put casts on my legs for my first year and it was accepted as the same *mystery illness* that had caused problems with my mother. In 1995, my mother walked into her doctor's office and told them to tell her what was causing her suffering or she would kill herself. Luckily for all of us, they diagnosed her with what Ehlers-Danlos Syndrome Type 3, now known as hypermobility EDS. Once she was diagnosed, it became obvious that this same condition had been causing my issues. I was evaluated and found to have mitral valve prolapse, and other than getting an echocardiogram every year or two, I wasn't really exposed to doctors myself. My mother went through a lot during that time and I saw what happened to her. Sometimes the surgeries worked and sometimes they only made it harder to keep her from committing suicide. The one constant was more bracing and less activity.

I learned about EDS by caring for my mother, myself, and through countless hours spent reading. My father was the only one who allowed me to do anything but he didn't know about EDS. Everyone else in my life kept me from moving or injuring myself at any cost. I was taken out of gym class and not allowed to play outside. I worked out in secret but it wasn't enough; never enough. One day I lost half a molar playing floor hockey and I couldn't hide exercising any more.

I left home fairly young and did alright for years until I was placed on bedrest during my second pregnancy. I obeyed my doctor's orders and, although my son is worth it, my life changed. Coming back from an extended period of inactivity is without a doubt the hardest thing I have ever done. I know it is a long journey, but I can feel that I am more than what my genetic mutations want me to be.

Since diagnosis and over the six years of going downhill fast, I learned much:

- Everything is equal.
- Find the joy in every second you can because you're going to go through it anyway.
- Never give up, because you never know the next time you'll be happy to be alive.
- Everyone who has any kind of trauma or loss has to go through the grieving process, but sometimes we have to do it again and again, and that's all right.
- Techniques like Mindfulness Based Stress Reduction can help to relax you both physically and emotionally, find peace and acceptance, and it can even lessen your pain and reduce stress.
- When you feel like someone doesn't understand, they probably don't, but that doesn't mean they don't wish they could.
- Trust your body and listen to what it tells you.

I am still in what I would call the beginning of my story, but even not knowing how it will end, I can tell you that there is always the strong probability of happiness, strength, and adventure in a truer meaning than you could have ever felt otherwise. You just have to do it.

WRITTEN BY SERINA ELYSE CASWELL

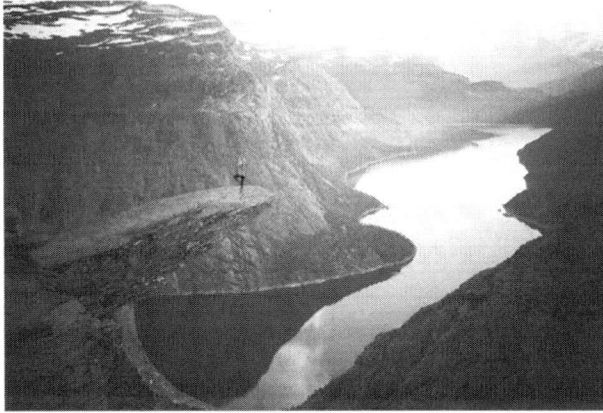

One day at a time –this is tough enough. Do not look back and grieve over the past for it is gone; and do not be troubled about the future, for it has not yet come. Live in the present, and make it so beautiful it will be worth remembering. – Unknown

A Hope and Prayer

In 1998, I married my hero, David. We lived a typical military life where our time together was made exceptionally more special by the deployments that separated us. We loved one another and desired nothing more than to grow our family. We were blessed with two beautiful children and looked forward to more. The traditional method of having children didn't work for us after our first two and we embarked upon the journey of In Vitro Fertilization (IVF) to make our dreams a reality. As we started the process, David received orders for his third tour in Iraq. Even without him home, we continued forward on a hope and a prayer that this treatment would be successful.

On the day of my first treatment, a woman I met through a fertility group surprised me. I walked into the waiting area to find Shelby waiting patiently with a yellow duck and a box of candy eggs as a gesture of hope that we would have success. She knew that my husband was deployed and didn't want me to go through the process alone. I was immeasurably thankful for her company and support. After the treatment was finished, I was told we had a 14-day wait before a blood test would be done to determine if it was successful. On bated breath, I waited.

After a mere seven days, I became extremely ill. Dr. B. ordered labs, including a pregnancy test. It was in the words, "You're pregnant!" where coping with the nausea became bearable. I was sent for an ultrasound and not only did we find one child, but two! Dr. B. was concerned about Baby B because the sac was small and there was very little fluid inside. He told me not to rush out and purchase two of everything because I would only bring one child home. In spite of his disheartening news, I reminded him that Baby B would be a fighter and I had hope that God would not bring us to this point for us to lose one.

As my pregnancy continued, we faced more complications with both Baby A and Baby B. My health suffered, too. While my husband was on guard duty in Iraq, a friend of his called to see how we were doing. I was excited to share the news that we were blessed with a boy and a girl. His comrades couldn't wait to share and announced the joyous news to the platoon. It was a mere 6 weeks later when my doctor made the request for my husband to return early from his tour to aid me as I could no longer handle the care of our entire family without his help. At 33 weeks, Baby A was in distress and we could no longer wait to deliver. I had an emergency caesarian section, delivering Noah, Baby A, at 5 pounds, 9 ounces and Hope, Baby B, at 2 pounds 9 ounces. In spite of a three-pound difference in weight, Hope's health was far better than predicted.

We knew that Hope would likely have health issues as a child and true to the course, she was slow to crawl and walk. She simply didn't thrive. Physically, she was weaker and her immune system couldn't handle a simple cold. At two, we transferred to Hawaii. A year had passed and our new pediatrician was concerned. Hope wasn't able to climb onto exam tables, pedal a tricycle, would fall often, and suffered many nose bleeds per day. She was noted to be like a "Gumby doll." We began seeing various specialists including occupational and physical therapists, neurologists, and rheumatologists. With each specialist we saw, they found something that led us to the next and back around again. After a years' time, we finally saw a geneticist and Hope was initially diagnosed with Ehlers- Danlos Syndrome, hypermobility type.

It's been 18 months since we left Hawaii for Georgia. The last year has been tough for Hope with three hospitalizations and one surgery. Her type of EDS is challenging because of her cardiac involvement and tissue fragility. Our new specialists and her pediatrician believe she has the vascular form and we will receive test results very soon. The list of diagnoses and medications continues to grow. We know that with the complications Hope has, her life and ours could change in an instant. Through it all, we've learned that our lives are not determined by physicians, but rest in God's hands. At each juncture in our journey, we have had exactly what and who we need; friends reaching out unexpectedly, family relationships strengthening, insightful doctors who gave us knowledge and understanding, and Hope has a brother with the greatest of strength who lives to encourage and support her. What we've gained is far less than watching the perseverance of Hope having hope.

Our bright-eyed little girl who has likely never known a day without pain or fatigue accepts this life of hers with grace, dignity, and a love of each moment like none we've known before. She dreams of the day when she can teach others delicate moves across gym mat or dance as a princess. It is on a hope and a prayer that she can see these dreams a reality.

AS TOLD BY DAWN MARIE BEALS

Strong and Courageous

After 42 years, I was finally given a diagnosis for my health issues, in May of 2012, by of ALL people, my psychiatrist! He diagnosed me the first time I saw him after reviewing my history, examining and talking to me because he has EDS himself. In his 30 years of practicing, I am the only person he has ever diagnosed with EDS. Up until then I thought I just had fibromyalgia, which was agreed upon by my family doctor and two rheumatologists. Several months later, I went to Tulane University Hospital (a teaching hospital) in New Orleans for a second opinion – and a more official diagnosis since people think you are crazy for saying you were diagnosed with a rare genetic connective tissue disorder by your SHRINK!

At that appointment, my EDS diagnosis was confirmed. A new diagnosis of mitral valve prolapse was made by a highly respected rheumatologist as well as a room of 5 medical students whom requested I perform my contortionist's circus tricks. I did not mind at all because they needed to know what Ehlers-Danlos Syndrome looks like beyond the medical book pictures. Anytime that I can be an advocate for EDS I am glad to do so. I have an upcoming appointment in 2 weeks with a geneticist at Oschner's in New Orleans to (hopefully) rule out vEDS (vascular type of EDS), which is the most deadly form.

I was born on January 1, 1971 in Monroe, LA. Shortly after birth, I was relinquished for adoption. I had the blessing of being adopted by the most amazing, loving, and dedicated Christian parents. I was raised with a brother who is 10 years older and their biological son. I have had joint and body pain as long as I can remember. My momma always told me it was growing pains. As a child I would fall asleep crying from pain, I vividly recall thousands of times, momma or daddy placing my legs in between theirs as in a scissor hold, keeping my legs completely still until I could finally doze off. The heat, stillness, and pressure somehow helped the pain enough to allow me to fall asleep. As an infant and child, I had numerous ear, urinary tract and kidney infections. Many infections were so severe that I had to be hospitalized. I also wore leg and ankle braces, corrective shoes and ankle-foot orthoses (AFO) as a toddler and child. I was also born tongue-tied and had a frenulectomy as a baby. I have had frequent sprains, strains, and pulled muscles from the simplest activities my entire life. Since my teens, I have had numerous kidney stones, all have had to be surgically removed because I have malformed ureters as well as a misshapen kidney. My gallbladder was also attached to my liver. I never knew it was not normal for joints to come out of place until I was grown. Every one of my joints hyperextend… some of them sublux while others completely dislocate with ease.

I've been very active my entire life until the last year. I began ballet, tap, jazz and acrobatics at age three through thirteen and loved it. During the summers through my teen years, I taught swim lessons and baton lessons with my mom while she was out on break from teaching. I began gymnastics when I was ten until age 14 when I fell on my head while doing back handsprings because my elbow popped out of place and I fractured my neck. I was also a cheerleader in my teen years. Looking back, I sometimes wish that I had done none of those activities because I know they contributed to the havoc on my body, but had I not done them, I would have missed out on a so-called normal childhood. I also wouldn't be the person I am today. But I do know all of those years of abuse to my joints, muscles, tendons, ligaments, and bones are a major reason that I have non-stop pain now.

Living a life with EDS is extremely hard. I honestly think no one understands what we endure. I would not wish this pain on the devil. I often describe my regular everyday pain as feeling as if I am being drawn and quartered – as if I am being stretched from my head to my feet in awful abnormal ways causing burning pain in the joints and muscles. This is a pain that never goes away, ever. I always have muscles that hurt or are sprained, so, of course, this causes additional pain. Then there is the feeling like my head is a fifty-pound bowling ball sitting on my shoulders due to cervical instability issues. This instability causes at least 20 headaches a month and these are not the normal run-of-the-mill headaches; they are excruciating and sometimes last days. This instability along with falling so much has caused my entire spine from my brain stem to my tail bone to give me nearly constant agony. I have urinary retention causing my bladder to often feel as though I have been kicked in the gut; causing me to double over just to be able to walk. I have gastrointestinal issues like IBS, reflux, and nausea after eating – as well as having stomach and diaphragm spasms that feel like an elephant sitting on me blocking my airway. I have an extremely hard time regulating my body temperature. I will be freezing in my extremities while pouring sweat from my head and torso... When I get up from sitting, my ankles are stiff, but my knees and hips are loose like noodles, leading to subluxation or dislocating my knees and/or hips. Sometimes, this leads to me falling.

It takes a physical therapist's mind plus an EDSers agility to know how to move without crumbling, stumbling or falling with each step or popping a knee, hip or even rib out of joint. I dislocate wrists from pulling covers up in bed; pop ribs out of place or dislocate my shoulders by just rolling over in bed and by pulling a shirt over my head. But this is all that I know, so it has become my way of life – my own normal. A life I would never wish upon anyone.

After finally being diagnosed, I have had the privilege of meeting hundreds of other Zebras. These people are the most kind and understanding humans on the planet. I do not know where I would be without my herd of Zebra friends. There are many times that I do not think I can endure and go on with this all-over, never-ending pain; but there is always a Zebra or a few Zebras that help me through the most painful times. I could never thank them enough for that.

I have been unable to work since March 2014, due to pain that causes severe insomnia, fibromyalgia, attention deficit disorder, myofascial pain, degenerative disc and joint disease, osteoarthritis, cervical instability, migraines, cluster headaches, depression and anxiety - all of which I know intimately and are caused by EDS! I have applied for social security disability and am awaiting a court date. I'll keep on fighting because I know no other way to be. My goal is to raise awareness and be an advocate for Ehlers-Danlos Syndrome so that everyone knows about EDS. Your child may have it and you NEED to know! I also hope, that through awareness, that one day there may be a cure for this dreaded, painful condition. It is difficult living with this disorder when you look normal, but inside you are far from normal. Looks can most surely be deceiving. My own family and most friends do not understand. I am not sure why God chose me to endure this battle, but I do know that I am stronger than I look and He will always pull me through. I am certain that those living with EDS are not weak in soul or mind.

Be strong and courageous. Do not fear or tremble before them, because the LORD your God will be the one who keeps on walking with you – he won't leave or abandon you. Deuteronomy 31:6

WRITTEN BY BOBBETTE PRIEST JANSSEN

I am a 44-year old Christian wife and mom to three sons Jake 24, Colton 18 and Samuel 6. I am my sons' biggest fan and supporter of their year-round sports and active lives. My sons keep me going along with my family, friends and, of course, my Heavenly Father above. I am currently unable to work due to my health conditions.

Since I was adopted at 21 days old, I have no idea where my Ehlers-Danlos came from or it was a random gene mutation. I am currently in the process of reuniting with my biological family as of late 2014. I have the most loving Christian parents who adopted me and raised me with a brother 10 years older than me. I also have a biological sister from my birth father who is 23 months younger than me as well as a biological brother from my birth mother who is a 23 months younger than me.

I enjoy all sports, going to church, shooting guns, nature, reading, surfing the Internet and social media, talking, watching Netflix and making others happy.

PERSPECTIVE

The only thing you sometimes have control over is perspective. You don't have control over your situation. But you have a choice about how you view it.
– Chris Pine

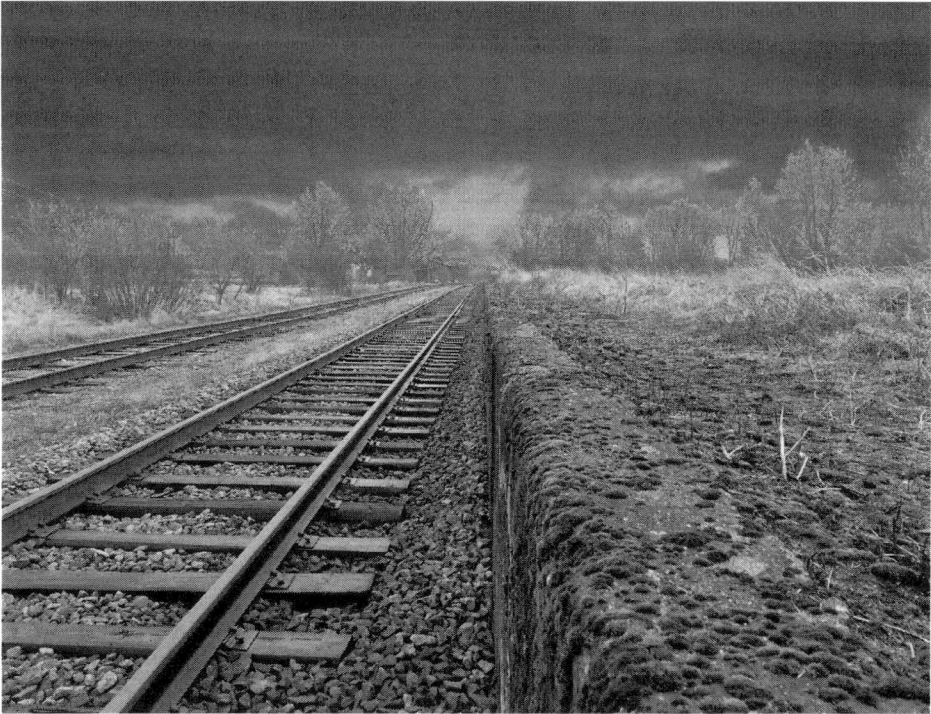

EDS

Entire photo series provided by Meghan Newsom as a showcase of hypermobility with Chris West's permission. Visit **MNewsomPhotography.com** for more about Meghan's photography. Some photographs are available only in print and digital color editions.

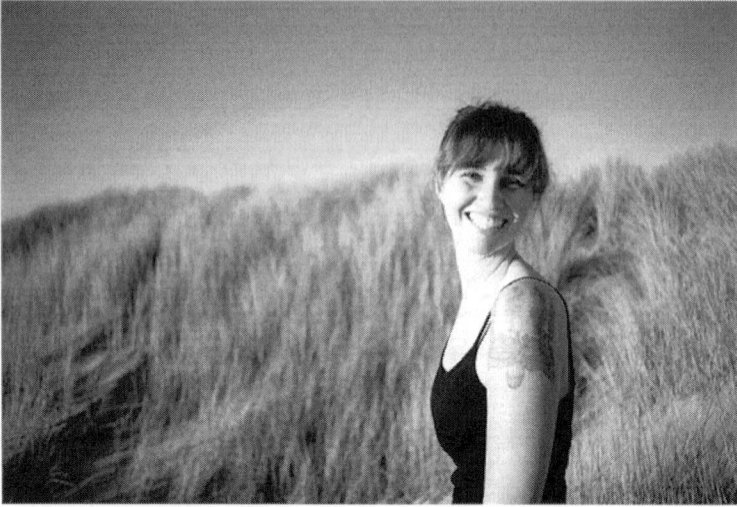

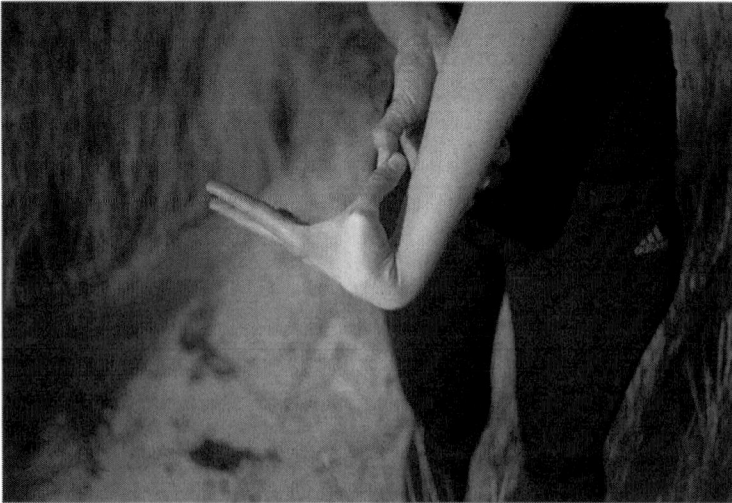

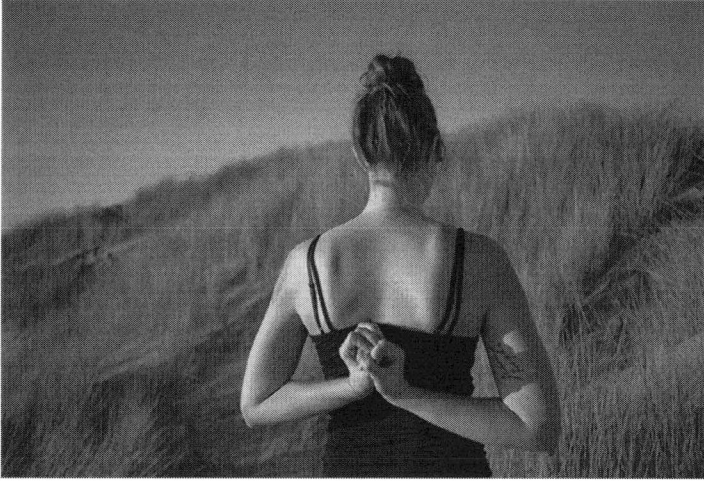

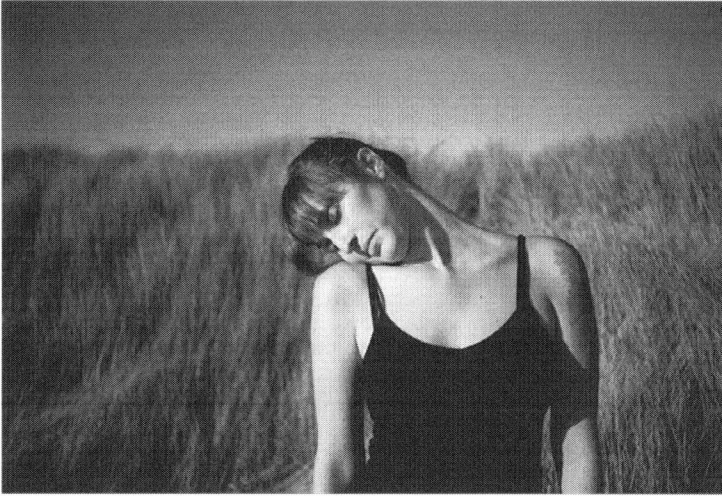

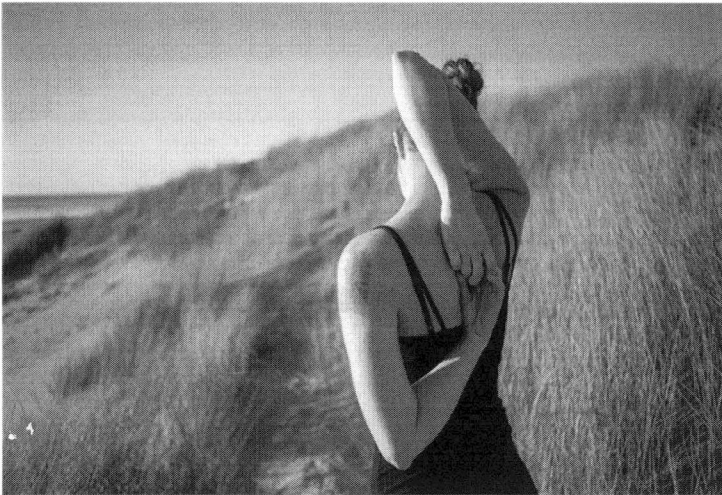

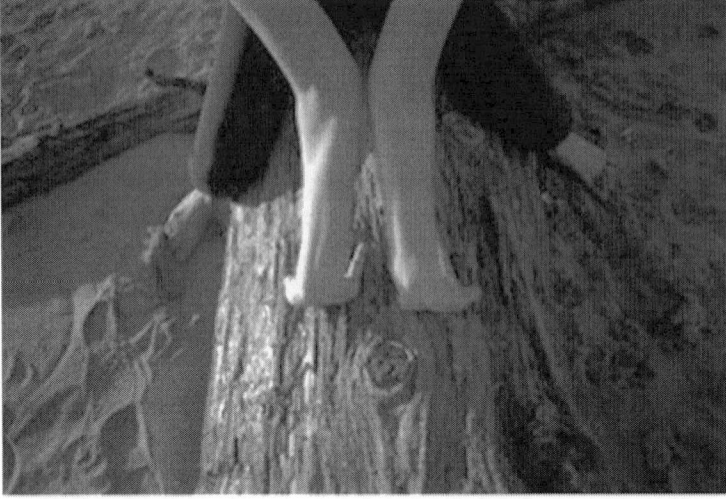

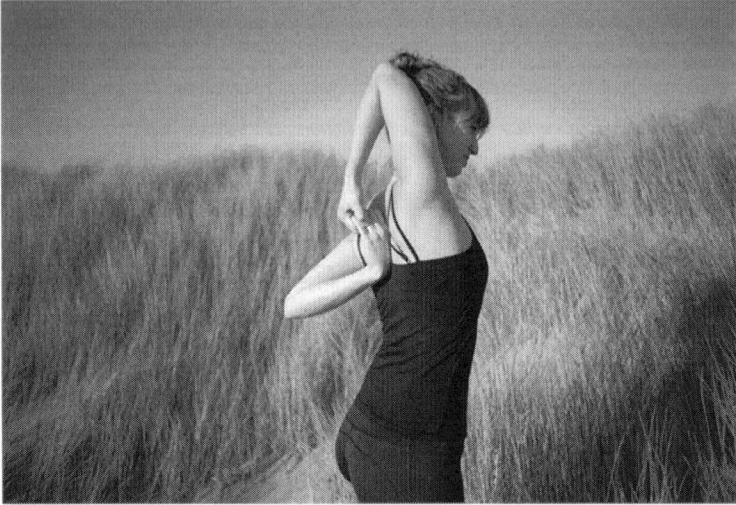

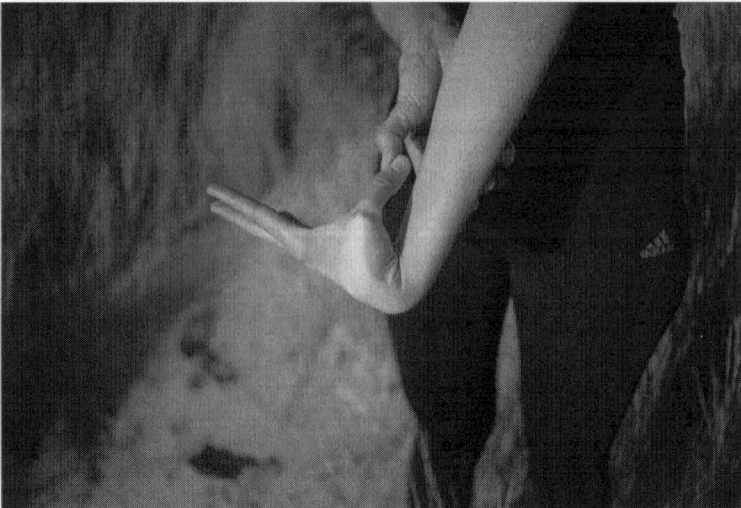

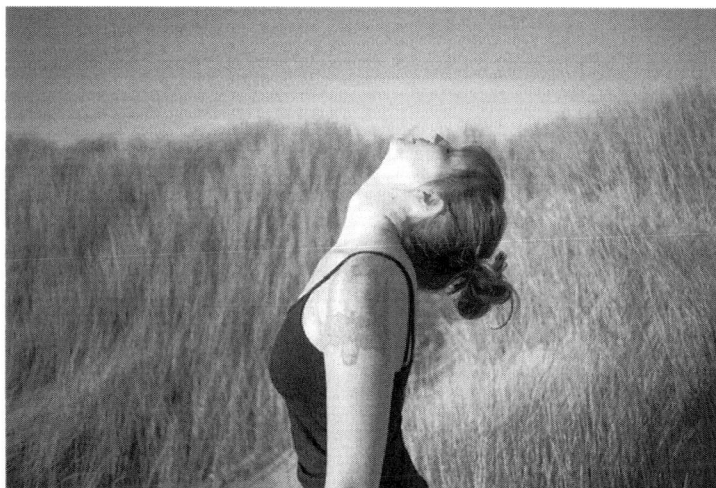

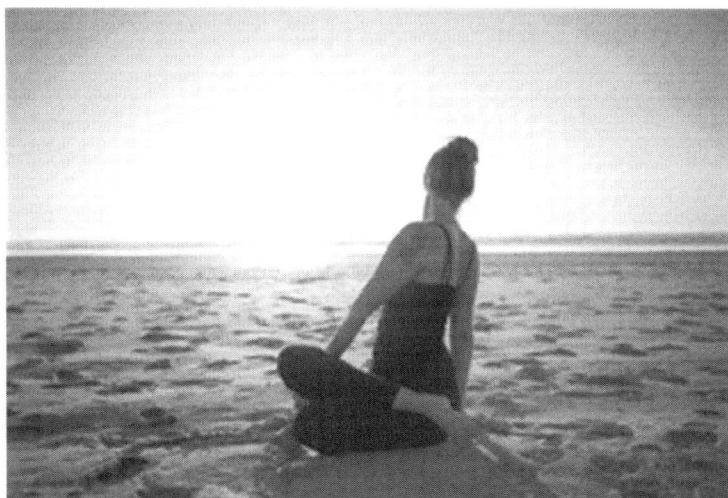

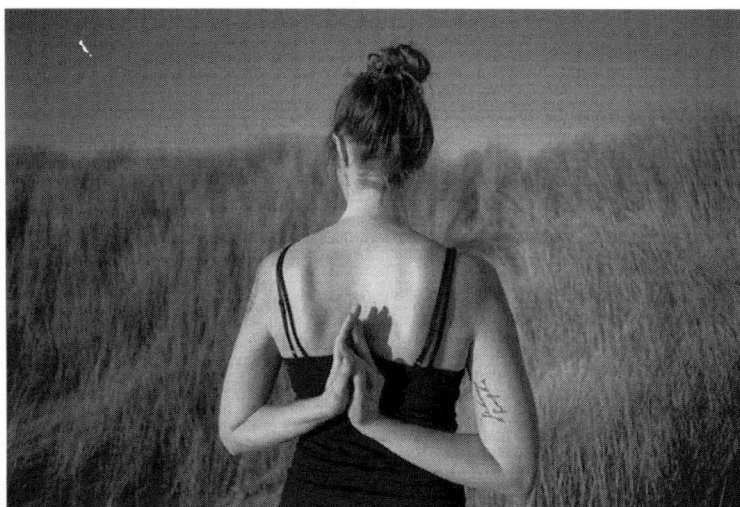

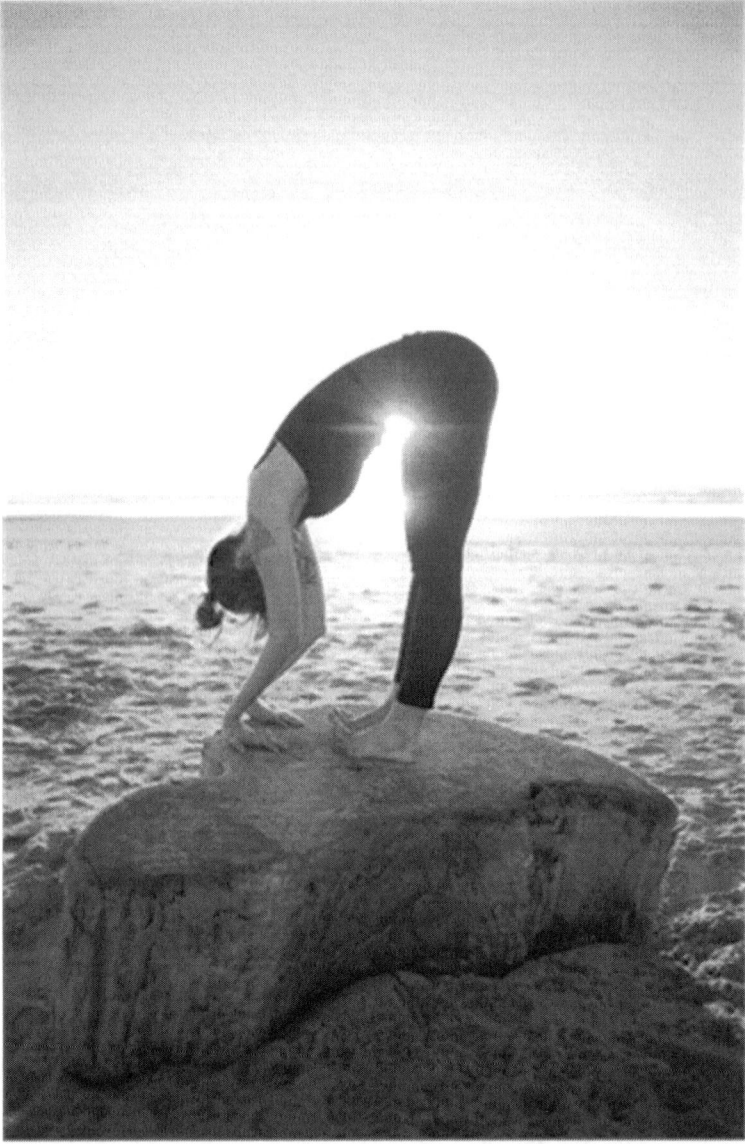

Unlocking the Doors

I was diagnosed with EDS hypermobility type (type III) in 2013 when I was 34. I've always known that I have joint hypermobility but it started causing issues when I was in my early twenties.

When I was 17, I started working with people with profound intellectual and physical disabilities. They brought out the best in me. They couldn't talk, but allowed me to talk for them. They couldn't eat, drink, or bathe themselves, but they were comfortable with me doing that for them. Their smiles put a smile on my face and in my heart. Soon after I started working, I found myself with joint pain and unstable wrists. The doctor told me to find another job because I shouldn't push a wheelchair or lift a client with them. It took a while before I actually changed jobs and it broke my heart when I did. I really thought I was meant for this job... I really loved helping others!

A few years later, I became a mother. I have two beautiful daughters who are totally worth the extra pain during and after the pregnancies. At the time I didn't know the extra pain was going to stay and I didn't know that my youngest daughter inherited EDS from me.

The greatest challenge in my health is coping with the deterioration. I used to dance, ride my bike, and walk for hours. Now I can hardly walk for 10 minutes. In the past 15 years, I have had to give up many of the things I love. It was like someone hit the brakes and I stood still while everyone else just continued without me. I couldn't raise or care for my kids the way I wanted and I was no longer able to do the job I loved so much. I felt useless. It made me sad to see options disappear and the doors closing in front of me.

There have been many changes because of my health after my diagnosis, but these changes are still not complete. At first, I continued being the young, wild, impulsive, and perfectionist me. I wanted to do it all and I wanted to do it right. I knew I had to give up some things at some point, but I didn't want it to be then. I wanted to keep up with everybody else, do my job just as well (or perhaps even better) as others, be able to go out and dance like my friends, and be the perfect mother, wife, sister, daughter, friend, etcetera. I didn't want anybody to notice what was wrong with me and I wouldn't talk about the pain because I didn't have a diagnosis. I was able to think that there wasn't anything really wrong with me.

I reached a point when I needed more and more wine to numb the pain and to push myself beyond my physical limits. It was time to take myself seriously. I went to a psychologist and sought therapy. I met with a rheumatologist and a geneticist. I was finally diagnosed with Ehlers-Danlos Syndrome and was ordered to have physiotherapy and occupational therapy.

Eventually, I became more peaceful. I knew I didn't have to be perfect any more. I accepted that it's okay to not do some things because there is a reason. I'm more forthcoming about EDS with others which has made me realize how blessed I am with the family and friends that surround me. They don't see me as the useless, incapable person I saw – but appreciate me for who I am, what I have (and do) accomplish even with EDS. They are willing to help wherever they can and I'm grateful.

My diagnosis and the change in my physical health have helped me to take a different perspective on my purpose. "When one door closes, another opens." When I stopped working with people with disabilities I started studying pedagogy and became a teacher. Now I can share my passion for those with disabilities with my students and spark passion in them.

I once read a poster from "Loesje" that said something like: "I used to think my limitations were my limits." It's true. I used to believe they were. Instead of giving up, my limitations motivated me to look further and made me discover other talents and ways to live a life with passion. I don't know what the future holds, but I do know that I will always find a way to adapt and make the most out of each day.

There are many turning points when you have Ehlers-Danlos Syndrome. Each time you are forced to give something up or accept something you don't like, you change. I changed when I had to give up a job that I loved, accept that I couldn't do everything on my own, face the reality of being diagnosed, and purchase a wheelchair. With each pivotal moment, I thought doors were closing, but instead discovered great blessings including teaching, family, friends, and encouragement. Some of these doors opened themselves, but when they didn't, I had to find the key or ring the bell. I wasn't willing to give up – and you shouldn't either.

The greatest lesson I learned is that I have a syndrome that doesn't kill me. It makes me stronger on a different level and I'll always have tools that make life that much better.

WRITTEN BY JACQUELINE VAN KUILENBURG

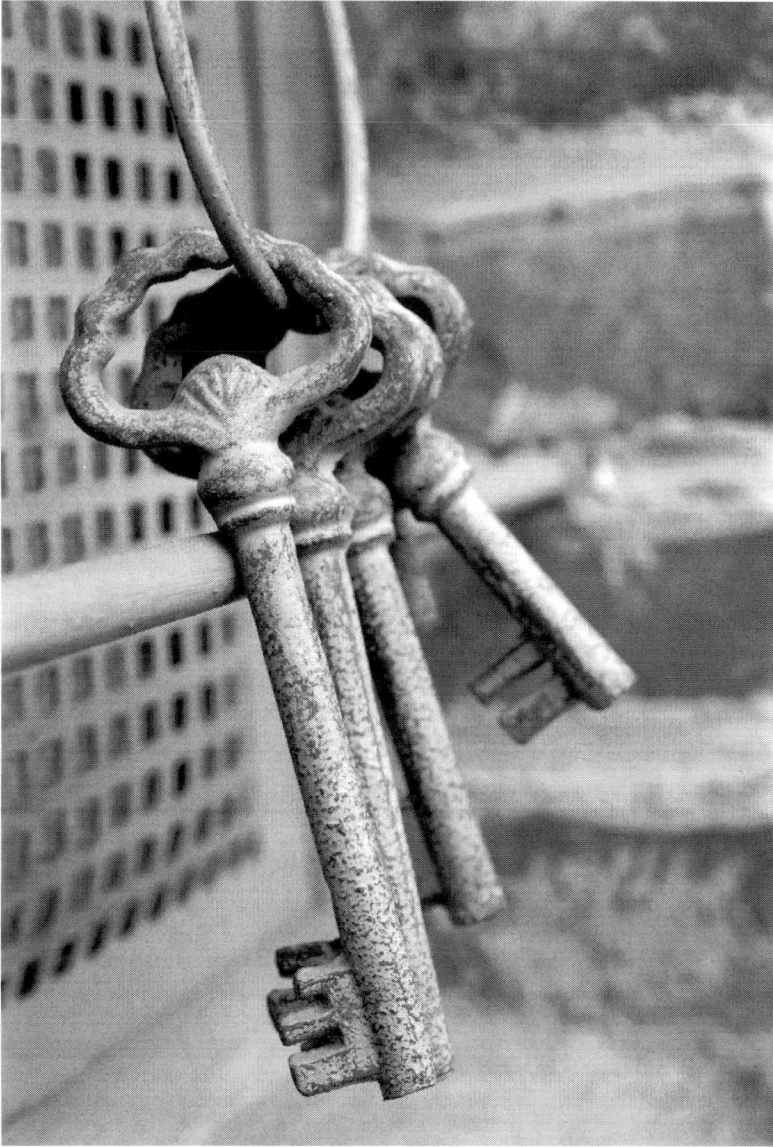

Married to EDS

My first reaction to the diagnosis of Classical Ehlers-Danlos Syndrome for my wife was shock and then the questions started to race through my head. What the hell did you just say? What is that? What does this mean? Does it affect her life expectancy? How will this affect her short-term and long-term? Does our little boy have this? It didn't take long to figure out that this was a "rare" condition/syndrome. I believe that the first numbers that I read was 1 in 200,000 people have the syndrome. That was reassuring, not! The information available via GOOGLE was not in the least bit encouraging. Then I got to the classification of Vascular Ehlers-Danlos Syndrome. The prognosis for these unfortunate people was so-so. Terrible story after terrible story littered the Internet. It was overwhelming.

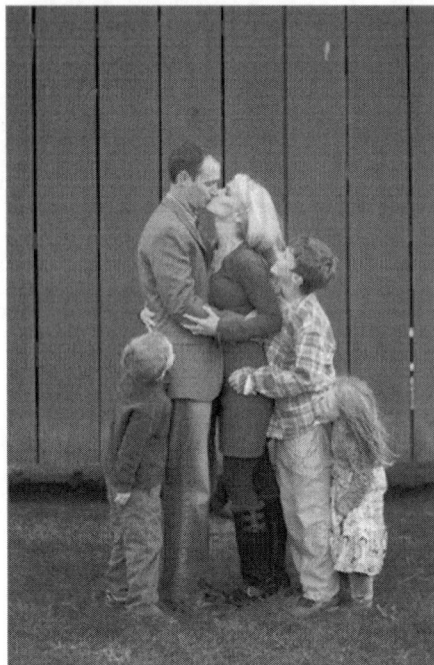

It was shortly after the birth of our first son that Kendra was diagnosed, approximately 10 months later. The pregnancy was very difficult on her, which also was complicated by the recent loss of her mom (10 days after we found out that we were expecting) and her demanding job in pharmaceutical sales. I knew pregnancy could take a toll on women; however the back, hip and leg pain seemed to be out of control. She suffered from dislocations, horrendous chronic pelvic pain and many other ailments that are common in EDS patients. The pregnancy and the cutback in her normal workout routine was enough to send her into a downward spiral and resulted in brachial plexitis in both shoulders due to muscle spasms and swelling at the end of her pregnancy. The pain was unbearable and there was nothing that could be done for this kind of pain during pregnancy. For the last 3 weeks of her pregnancy, Kendra would lay in one position on our bed, the only position that gave some relief to the nerve pain in her shoulder, and also was a position that didn't exacerbate the constant Braxton-Hicks contractions, which caused early dilation and effacing. The baby had to *cook* for just a bit longer in order to allow his lungs to develop.

I want to share a little history on Kendra pre-children Kendra was very active, loved working out and could be talked into even the craziest things outdoors. We lived an active life filled with hiking, backpacking, camping, rock climbing and anything to do on the water. It was not infrequent that Kendra would stay up to all hours of the night to get a workout in. She loves her DVD workout videos – in the early days it was the FIRM videos. The point is, Kendra was in excellent shape. The pregnancy, which led to the additional laxity of her joints, caused terrible chronic pain. Massage seemed to help, however the result of long pressure filled massages left her looking like I beat her with a broom handle.

We are fortunate enough to live in an area of the country that has the best medical care in the world. Living in between Washington, DC and Baltimore, MD, we had access to the best MDs in the world; including Johns Hopkins, University of Maryland, Georgetown University, George Washington University, and NIH. Surely we would be able to get the care that Kendra needed and the roadmap that we both were seeking. To my surprise, she did get diagnosed; however the information and the treatment for the syndrome were not all that well-known. Let me say, the physicians that Kendra first saw did not understand EDS as it was not well-known, nor well understood by those who did know enough to diagnose it. The guidance and direction that Kendra received was to go on long-term disability and start a steady dose of narcotics and sedatives to cope with the pain.

Did I mention that Kendra was very active? This direction was not taken lightly and the quest for knowledge started. Against doctors' orders, Kendra started the long and lonely journey to get herself back to a thriving lifestyle. We had a beautiful little boy that needed his mother, we needed to decide on whether or not to have more children, and make a decision on social security disability or for Kendra to find a way to work and help support our family while also taking care of herself. Kendra's determination was unrelenting. Almost 2 years after the birth of our first son, Kendra was back to her strong active lifestyle. She coped with the pain and simply pushed on.

Kendra would often tell me that she would lose muscle in a very quick time period if she did not workout. At first I thought she was crazy and was just playing the card so she had a little alone time. Looking back now, Kendra had already figured out a major component of living and thriving with EDS ...working out! By building and toning all the major muscles and core muscles required to dance and do her videos, Kendra was creating stability within her joints. This stability that she created allowed her to thrive until she became pregnant with our second little boy.

The cycle repeated itself. Post-pregnancy Kendra was a hot mess. She was in excruciating pain and found herself in the midst of another downward spiral. The recovery time from the second pregnancy was faster because Kendra knew what she needed to do - exercise and begin to regain her strength and energy! And then we found out that we were pregnant with baby #3. This news came as both a shock and a surprise, something we wanted but just not quite yet. The back-to-back pregnancies proved to be very tough on Kendra physically, as well as on our family life and her thriving medical sales business.

As many EDS patients suffer from a variety of ailments, Kendra was not the exception to this rule. Chronic pain, migraine headaches, slow gastric motility, numerous debilitating pelvic issues (i.e., pelvic congestion), chronic fatigue; the list goes on. What amazed me, was that many of her specialists never connected the dots with all her symptoms. They would remember a page in a textbook that they reviewed in med school and that was the extent of their knowledge base on EDS. I lost count of the number of times that Kendra would start educating her doctors on EDS. That was eye opening and very scary.

Kendra has dealt with the pain and the numerous comorbid diagnoses by remaining active, focusing on the positive, working for herself and helping the EDS community by speaking at the University of Maryland genetics department to first-year medical students, volunteering with EDNF to answer help line questions, and starting a second business to help patients with EDS find information and resources they need to live as healthy a life as possible with EDS and now... this anthology.

Looking back over the years, this syndrome has affected every part of our lives; from finances, our relationship, mental attitude, sleep, exercise, parenting, and what our family eats. We have adapted and adjusted our lives to make the syndrome tolerable for Kendra and for our children. This is not the *woe is me* portion of my story, but rather the part that states the obvious. People with EDS need to adjust their lifestyles and it is all encompassing. We had to work through many family members not understanding that EDS was a condition that could cause so many issues or *that much pain.* It was even more difficult for some because Kendra didn't look *sick* – she was called beautiful, healthy, and told that people would give their right arm to look like her. They couldn't *see* her struggle.

It's also been quite obvious how *not so rare* EDS really is. Since Kendra was diagnosed, we've had some of our closest friends and family also get diagnosed, including my best friend Kyle, whose story is also in this book. What are the chances? Pretty high, now that we know that EDS is not rare, but rarely diagnosed and often misdiagnosed as numerous other conditions or just completely ignored.

Good nutrition, exercise, and a positive outlook are the pieces to the puzzle that started to bring clarity to living and striving with EDS for our family. In fact, it's imperative.

To those of us, like myself, that love and care for someone with EDS, my words of encouragement are things can get better. At the end of the day, it's up to the individual with the condition to make the required changes. It's my role/our role to support and encourage our significant other/s to continue to climb out of the downward spiral. In addition to supporting Kendra and becoming a great masseuse, I have learned that I must also support 3 children that are also showing various signs and symptoms of this condition. Talk about motivation… It's critical that I understand EDS and help create the environment that supports each of my children's blind spots pertaining to EDS. Over time, our three children will learn about EDS and the daily choices that they need to make to thrive and succeed in living with EDS. Be courageous and support the ones that you love with EDS. The journey constantly changes and there are always obstacles that need to be overcome. With a strong support system, my hope is that Kendra is able to continue to live and thrive while living with EDS and all others living with EDS find that same safe haven.

WRITTEN BY BRIAN MYLES

Brian & Kendra have been married for just over 12 years and have been together since the end of their senior year in high school. Brian is a manager in the medical device field and has 3 beautiful children with Kendra. He is an avid fisherman, loves to vacation with his family, watch the Capitals, cook with his brother-in-law Dan and just completed his first half-Ironman.

Professional photographs by Helen John Photography.
HelenJohnPhotography.com

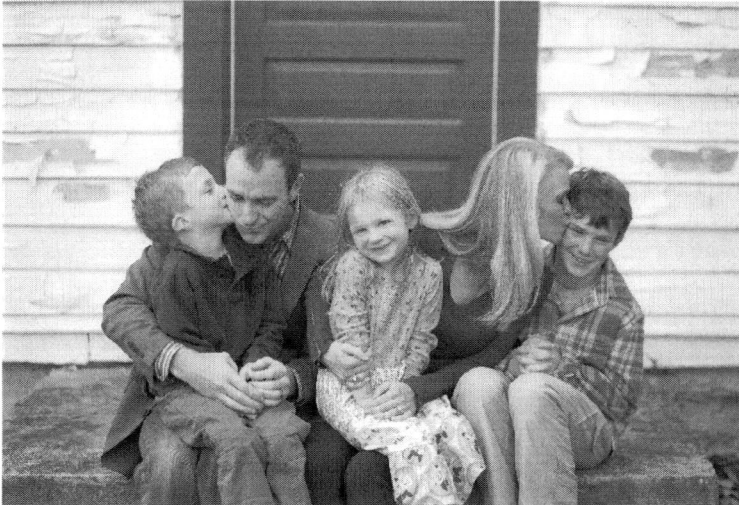

Dear Teacher

Editorial Note: This post originally appeared on Sarah Wells' blog. The only changes made include converting words from British to American English and photos were removed.

Writing my latest blog entry has been an emotional and cathartic experience. It is based on supporting my three children through their whole school experience so far. Being a mum to children with physical needs is much more emotionally draining than having those needs yourself. It's much longer than I planned but once I started writing I has so much to say.

My children have EDS (HMS) or CMT or a combination of the two but I think that teachers and parents of many children with special educational or medical needs will relate to elements of my blog.

Dear teacher...

I appreciate how hard it is for you, I am a former teacher. Thirty children in your class; low ability, more able, English as an additional language, disadvantaged pupils, those with special needs like ADHD or autism and then my child in their own unique category, with a medical need that wears a cloak of invisibility.

In my family there is Charcot Marie Tooth disease, a peripheral neuropathy affecting the motor and sensory nerves in the arms and legs causing weakness and sensory loss, one of my 3 children has been diagnosed with this. We also have Ehlers-Danlos Syndrome, a problem with the body's connective tissue, the glue that holds you together. All of the children have symptoms of this to some extent. Ranging from bendiness to pain, fatigue, gastrointestinal problems, easy bruising, skin issues and dizziness. Both conditions are genetically passed on.

What these conditions have in common is that you can't easily see them. Unless a child has had a dislocation and is wearing a brace or you happen to glance at them when they are 'w' siting or have their body in another strange position then they will look like any other child in the class.

You can't see the orthotics in their shoes trying to align their feet and ankle bones as they walk but you may notice that as the day and week goes on their legs don't really hold them up any more and they fall and hurt themselves more often, or that you are sending home increasing amounts of letters about injuries.

You can't see the brace that they wear under their uniform to keep their shoulder in place but you may notice that they aren't as strong on their dominant side when they throw a ball because of their weakness after a dislocation. You won't see the knee supports they wear under their school trousers just to stop them aching so much by the end of a school day but you may notice them fidgeting in their seat more as the day goes on or as they try to change position when everything hurts.

You can't see that they become dizzy on standing (sometimes even sitting), you can't see that their blood pressure doesn't regulate correctly, particularly after lunch when their blood is needed to digest their food. You may notice that they need to drink more or they don't concentrate so much at certain times of the day.

You can't see their fatigue, it in itself has many different forms; where they wake up tired even though they are getting a good night's sleep, where their muscles don't have the energy to do a simple job, or when they can't think straight and their brain is "foggy." You won't really see my children be so physically exhausted that they are nauseous or vomit, we try hard to manage them so that it does not reach this extreme, but often it does. More often you may see them leaning on a chair, a doorway, a table because they find it hard to stand. You may see them slump over their desk for support because their body finds it tricky holding them in an upright sitting position. You may notice the dark, dark circles beneath their eyes even though they were in bed early every night this week. You might notice them get left behind when running in the playground because they can't keep up no matter how hard they try or them choosing to play positions on the football pitch where they don't have to run so much. When the fatigue is particularly bad you may even see a child choose not to join in with their friends because they are so tired, to choose to rest at playtime on their own.

You can't see pain, but you may see a fidgety child who can't seem to get comfortable in any position who rubs their joints or struggles getting up from the carpet. Or you may see them fall because their legs give way or their jaw get stuck momentarily as they yawn and it pop back into place.

While all of these things are invisible at first glance, for a good teacher, one who is in tune with the needs of the children in their class, if you look closely, you will see.

My children are confident, they are bright. They won't be the ones struggling with the work in class, they are switched on to the job that needs to be done. They will be making progress on the data sheets, but it is important that their condition is never allowed to get in the way of this. My children have developed many coping strategies and on the most part do not admit that they are in pain, they accept it as normality. One of my children, the one with the most needs, is super independent and determined. A quality I admire and would never like to change but I know it may seem that she doesn't need your help. She does.

What you may be unaware of is what goes on at home for my children. The fatigue is the trickiest thing to balance the meltdowns after school, the falls. Even when the fatigue is relentless getting to sleep can be really tricky because people with EDS or hypermobility make extra adrenaline. Once they get to sleep pain and cramp can disturb them at night adding to the fatigue the next day.

You won't know that we still have to use a buggy for our 5 year old or a scooter so that when she is tired she can be pulled. At home we do endless physio, this is really hard when everyone is tired at the end of a school day but so important to build stamina and stay strong. You won't see the gators tucked under the bed for stretching, the numerous gym balls dotted around the house or the designated drawer in the kitchen for therabands and hand putty. You won't realize all of the hospital appointments that the children attend both before and after school adding to the length of their day. In half a term one of my children attended 8 hospital, GP or physio appointments and I have had 7 lengthy phone calls with different professionals involved in their care.

You may not be aware how important stamina is for our children, taking part in sports is crucial. Please don't think that because they worked hard and got man of the match playing football for the school team that they are better now. What you don't see is the payoff for that reward, two days of severe pain and a week off of school recovering because symptoms have flared up. Is it all worth it? Yes. They are children and these memories are important.

Will we stop them attending a party at the weekend, playing football or even climbing trees at Go Ape? No. We plan, pace, limit the risks, brace where we need to and not relax for a minute but we will let them be children, have a go, sometimes fail and get up and try again and be prepared for the payoff later.

What you may not know is that as these conditions are genetic one of the parents will be affected. Usually painting on their smile and pretending that the pain, fatigue and autonomic dysfunction as well as daily dislocations and subluxations just aren't happening. After all there isn't time for all of that! Living with the conditions ourselves we understand the struggle to be 'normal' and we know that what they are experiencing is real. Remember, the most powerful thing you can say to a child with an invisible illness is... "I believe you."

I know that teachers want to do the best for my children, I can see it in their faces. I'm not blaming them or shaming them, the opposite in fact, I want to help them. I wonder if they have ever asked themselves at the end of a hard day; have I thought of everything? Could I have done more today? What can I do next? This may help to come at it from a different angle.

What can you do as a teacher to help my children? Take the time to learn, I know you are experienced and may have taught many children with special needs but every child is unique, including my children. Read their notes, ask questions of us as parents, of the SENCO, occupational therapists and physiotherapists involved in their care. Most importantly get to know my child and how their needs affect them in a school day and remember their condition may vary from day to day or even within the same day. Once you do get to know them then you will spot the signs of tiredness and pain much more easily, putting the adaptations and rest breaks in place will become much easier. We don't expect you to know it all, as parents we learn every day, since our children's symptoms started, we have read extensively about their conditions, we keep up to date with any developments and network with other parents. We spend the most time with them and are most definitely the experts in their care. Our knowledge and personal experiences may mean we appear over fussy and protective, but we fully understand the impact that bad management in childhood can have in later life; both with their bodies autonomic system and with damage to their joints.

You must accept that your teaching style or classroom organization may have to change. These may be simple things like; allowing them 5 minutes to stretch after a long assembly before they sit down in class to work, having their coat peg in a position where they won't be knocked by other children or sitting down for 2 or 3 minutes while you give the instructions to the class in PE before the task begins. However it may sometimes involve carefully pacing all their activities and planning in rest breaks to avoid them falling into a nasty cycle of fatigue. Please do not underestimate the impact that these changes can have on a child.

You will need to think ahead when planning school trips, outings, lengthy rehearsals and sports day. You have to carefully consider the impact that it may have on them including what extra support they will need in order to fully participate. When everything is planned and considered the knock on affects for their health later that day or week can be greatly minimized.

We will do our utmost to tell you if something different has happened at home or before school, if they have had an injury, are in a flare or are particularly fatigued.

Please make this easy to do, don't always tell us how bad their day has been at the end of a school day when they are listening. We try so hard as parents to give them a positive self-image and to be positive about their condition. While we need to know what has happened please consider what will be the best way to communicate by email, link book, text or telephone call.

You will need to communicate with the other professionals that are involved with our children from the lunch time assistants to other teachers, teaching assistants, the school nurse, physiotherapists and occupational therapists. We appreciate that you are all very busy but it is very difficult for us to become everyone's PA, ensuring open lines of communication between all parties. If you keep us regularly informed we will not keep bothering you for updates.

Please be flexible with homework, while our children are often competent enough for the tasks that you set, school is hard work for our children as they struggle to be 'normal' all day. This takes a lot of concentration and is very tiring. When our children get home from school, they are often exhausted and have to rest, it can be difficult to get them to do their homework. Remember that we often have physiotherapy or occupational therapy to do with our children in the evenings and at the weekends and they may have attended appointments as well. We value their school work, we do, after all our children will need to use their brains! However we also value the importance of them being children, attending clubs such as 'cubs' and 'swimming' outside school is important too. Keeping all the balls in the air can be hard work, requiring great skill.

It is common for children with health conditions to be affected emotionally. While my children are confident, don't let that confidence fool you, they are fully aware of their differences. My older child chooses not to discuss this with his friends, he doesn't want any undue attention but he understands that to manage this he has to communicate with the adults at school. This requires trust. My younger child is feeling left behind by the children in the playground, it bothers her. If these issues aren't managed well they will become compounded and will affect their work in school. Involve the children, put the *child* into a 'child-centered-approach', and talk to them.

We are trusting you with the most precious things in our lives to educate them and manage their care during school hours. As a teacher you are "responsible for the progress and development of all pupils" and with this privilege comes great responsibility. For those 6 hours a day we rely on your knowledge of our children and your skill of being able to recognize the subtle cues about their health. If you act on what you see by pacing, simple classroom adaptations, chill out time, hydration and changing position regularly you will help them to manage their condition and ultimately improve their health. Rather than the alternative, to sink deeper into a flare, become more fatigued or to have more injuries. All that has to be better for their education?

So much time and effort is spent dealing with our children's health it becomes important not to overlook their strengths, like all children they want to do well and they need your approval. There will be areas of the curriculum that they always find tricky, we know that, so when they are good at something please don't forget to give them their chance to shine! In the words of Magic Johnson "All kids need is a little help, a little hope and somebody who believes in them."

WRITTEN BY SARAH WELLS

I am a busy mum of three adorable children and a naughty French bulldog with the added bonus of Ehlers-Danlos Syndrome, Charcot Marie Tooth disease and the lovely symptoms of autonomic dysfunction throwing me a curve ball. I manage life wearing rose tinted glasses and a large glass of cup half full. I want to help others living with chronic illness or those who have children and are negotiating the slippery path between school, health and hospitals and to hopefully raise a little awareness along the way.

Follow Sarah's Blog: **mystripylife.blogspot.co.uk**

Spontaneous Genetic Mutation Lives On

(Q&A with Kristi Posival)

What type of EDS do you have and when were you diagnosed?

In 1979, I was a five-year old little girl two weeks away from starting kindergarten. It was the evening of August 16th, (my mother's birthday) and my parents had just returned home from a night out. I was sound asleep after a fun night with my favorite babysitter. A sudden commotion in the living room woke me. I left my room to find my father pacing and hiccupping uncontrollably. My mother was demanding to know what was wrong, but he wasn't able to speak. My father ended up collapsing in the kitchen. As he hit the floor his arm caught the metal cold air return, ripping his skin wide open. Blood pooled around my tiny toes as I stood over him. My mother was frantic on the phone with 911. When the ambulance arrived, my father was no longer breathing. There was a lot of yelling and movement but they said he was alive and strapped him to a gurney. My mom jumped in the ambulance with my father and they drove away. I stood in the summer darkness, crickets chirping, feeling the cool breeze on my skin alone in my pajamas with my father's dried blood between my toes. I have no idea how long I waited, less than five minutes but I still remember it is an eternity. Our neighbor came and grabbed some clothes for me. I spent the next three nights at her house. It was an eventful few days. I was given the top bunk in her son's bedroom. I should mention I sleep with my eyes open, so the first morning she came in to check on me and the whites of my eyes were showing with my pupils rolled back. She thought I had died and screamed, loudly! The shock scared me and I flew out of bed hitting the ceiling then the ground. I was left with a goose egg on my head and a nasty bruise on my side where I hit the floor. The next day I suffered my first bee sting and while I am not allergic the swelling was intense. On day three it was decided I should move on to the next neighbor's house. Things started well the first few nights, but tragedy struck again. We were playing ping-pong and I was on the father's team against his two sons. It was a competitive match and the father accidentally hit me in the face with the paddle resulting in a huge black eye. Time to move on. The third neighbor's house was fun. We played a lot in between my visits to the hospital. My father was in ICU the entire time and in 1979 children were not allowed. I did see him once though. My father was returning from another surgery so I waited by the elevator doors. As they opened I got to run alongside his hospital bed and hold his hand, until we hit the ICU doors, then I was forced to let go. I eventually moved on to a fourth neighbor's home. On the morning of September 1st my aunt picked me up and we headed to the hospital. My father had passed after several surgeries and fighting hard for 14 days. It was determined that his colon had perforated. He was 31 years old. During his autopsy they discovered Vascular EDS formerly known as Type IV. After the funeral my mother threw away all of his belongings. The only thing that remained was his spontaneous genetic mutation passed on to me.

Doctors were able to clinically diagnose me immediately and we waited almost a year for the results of the tissue biopsy. I was confirmed with the COL3A1 gene mutation in 1980. Oddly, I had to get retested in 2007 when doctors decided I was not what they considered EDS to be. The tissue biopsy came back positive, again, and the realization that many doctors have little understanding of this disease was confirmed, again.

What has been your greatest challenge in your health?

The lack of knowledge and awareness in the medical community is a monumental struggle. This lack of information makes it difficult to find helpful treatments, and also results in an adversarial experience with physicians.

After my initial diagnosis, I was told three things every year at my physical. "Be careful", "No gym class" and "I should never have children." Actually, the third thing didn't start until I was 12. I followed the doctors' requests for the most part, but still suffered a laundry list of injuries, bruises, dislocations and ruptured veins. I was left to figure out most of it on my own. I knew ice felt really good on veins that rupture. I taught my best friend how to pop my fingers back into place so we could keep playing. You know, the little things. I always thought one day I'll grow up and find a doctor who will help me, but the medical system just doesn't work that way. There are people studying the disease but the day-to-day needs are a challenge.

Most doctors are unfamiliar with EDS, are unaware of the various types (and the vascular type is its own beast) or if they have heard of it, but it is just the one page description in a medical textbook. This has created an atmosphere of distrust between medical professionals and me. For example, a decade ago I was in the ER because my foot was in severe pain. I assumed I fractured a bone but the test came back negative. I asked if they could just give me something for the pain over the weekend until I could get in to see my primary doctor (It was Friday night). The doctor called me a drug seeker to my mortified face, in front of three residents who wanted to meet someone with vEDS. Along these same lines, I recently saw the head of Pain Management at Johns Hopkins who accused me of the same thing – simply seeking drugs. (Last time I checked there wasn't a large demand on the street for cortisone injections.) There is a grey area as a patient because I know a lot about my condition and doctors don't always recognize the validity of my opinion. I tend to be assertive and matter of fact about why I see a doctor and what I want from them – I have 36 years of practice. It's not just pain doctors. I was in the ER a week before my colon perforated because I knew something was wrong. They miss-diagnosed my condition, released me, and I was back in the ER the following week having an emergency ileostomy. This type of situation isn't the exception; it's more the rule.

How have you changed because of your diagnosis?

Frankly, I don't remember a time when I didn't have a positive vEDS diagnosis. I have always known, which has advantages and disadvantages. The real feeling created from my diagnosis was that I was different. As a young child, I stood out in some way and that can be very lonely.

Kids recognized it immediately. For example, on the playground they would ask why my legs bent backwards when I stood straight. This turned into name calling, etc. As I got older bullying became the norm. The jocks in high school used to step on my heels to see if they could make me bleed. It worked, often. The isolation continues into adulthood in a more sophisticated manner. After college my priority was finding a job that offered health care. With a pre-existing condition in the '90s it was the only way to get health insurance. Something my roommates didn't have to worry about. Getting a new job and wondering how to disclose or if I *should* disclose my serious medical condition. Going on several dates with the same guy that I really liked who keeps asking about my many scars and bruises. Is it the third date I tell him the truth? How much do I disclose before he runs the other way? EDS continually reminds you you're different. Other people don't have to deal with that sort of crisis thinking in many aspects of their life. Should I ride in a car? Will the airbag break my arm or worse kill me? I have gas or maybe my colon is obstructed. No wait, my spleen ruptured. I run up the stairs, feeling out of breath. Am I tired or do I have another blood clot that ruptured and filled my lungs? We may be missing a layer of tissue but we have an added layer of uncertainty that is unknown to most people. An EDS diagnosis has an element of solitary confinement to it.

What is something you have overcome in your health?

This is a very difficult question to answer only because there are so many obstacles. Do I pick the time I cracked my head open and needed stitches, or the time I cracked my head open and needed staples? The time I severed my Achilles tendon while riding a bicycle with spiked pedals? The three different times I fractured my nose? Maybe the time in college when my quadricep muscle spontaneously ruptured causing me to permanently walk with a limp? (That was painful!) There are deep varicosities in my legs that started at age 19 and the pain still keeps me up at night at age 41. So many more to choose from but one of the scariest and most difficult challenges happened last year. February 6, 2014, I woke up around 5 am with a constant pain in my side. It was nothing I had felt before and while I had much worse pain over the course of my life there was something not right about this one. It was sharp and there was no reprieve. My husband took me to the ER around 8 am and by 1:30 pm they had determined my colon perforated, just like my father's had 35 years earlier. I had been told my entire life that the likelihood of my colon rupturing was high. The day it actually happened was such a whirlwind of emotions, but I was pumped full of morphine so I think I was handling it a bit better than my husband. We were frightened and this deep black hole of uncertainty rested over us with no light able to peak in. I was septic and required immediate surgery. The surgeon arrived and told us a good case scenario would be removal of part of my colon and a permanent ileostomy. It happened so fast. I signed some papers and kissed my husband goodbye. Neither one of us certain we would see each other again as they wheeled me down the hall to prep for surgery. I made it through and survived the successful ileostomy reversal 8 weeks later. I had a total of 150 staples and 21 days in the hospital between the two surgeries. I feel pretty damn lucky!

Another huge challenge I'd really like to share happened in 2006. I was invited to a dinner party and the hostess's cat attacked my right hand. I was left with a deep bite and several deep scratches. I went to the ER where a plastic surgeon was called in to consult and I was admitted to the hospital for "cat scratch fever." They aggressively cleaned the wound, along with strong liquid antibiotics to get rid of the infection. I was discharged after a few days and followed up with the plastic surgeon a week later. I could no longer move my fingers. Scar tissue had filled my hand and attached to my tendons so my fingers were stuck straight. This started a life-changing chain of events. Over the next 5 years, I underwent 5 hand surgeries including a flap and a skin graph, and years of occupational therapy. I'm an artist, love to paint and this was my dominant hand. I don't remember feeling more broken in my life. The final surgery was performed at Mayo Clinic in 2010. The doctor GREATLY improved my mobility. I continue to this day with occupational therapy and my hand cramps easily and often, but it is useable and I'm painting again.

Did you have a major turning point? If so, what was it and how did your life change?

Something happened in 1982 that put my life into perspective and has taken decades to fully grasp. I was 8; it had been 3 years since my father had passed. My mother was clinically depressed and stayed in bed most days. One night she told me to grab Tigger (my Siamese cat) and jump in the front seat of the car. I knew something was off because I NEVER got to sit in the front seat. She was quiet, her eyes red from crying. I did as she said and she joined me. We sat in the garage and she started the engine. The only thing she added was we are off to see Daddy. I knew that wasn't right. I knew he was gone. "I don't want to see Daddy." I cried as I opened the door and jumped out of that car. She turned off the engine. I ran to my room with Tigger and my mother called me selfish before I reached the door. For a long time, I thought she was right. My 8-year old mind thought it was selfish to prevent my mother from seeing my father again. Especially when she was so depressed. I was willing to do anything to help my "mommy" but I just didn't want to die. Of course, the reality is there is no selfishness in choosing to live. I wanted my life more than the promise of *seeing* my father again. I have tried to take that choice and live life to the fullest every day I can. I also recognized early on my mental capacity and strength is so much stronger than that of my body, and that's important – a strong mind can compensate mightily for a weak body.

High school was terrible, but by college I was seeing a real future on the horizon. I graduated from college and moved to Chicago to start my life. I worked hard and had some okay-jobs and then a great job. I made friends. I stayed out late. I dated. I sought out the right health care professionals. I spent an unbelievable amount of money on my teeth! (They like to break.) The main life lesson though, was that I learned how to take care of myself and I was good at it. I had been doing it on my own for so long without realizing it, so putting it into practice felt amazing. Eventually I fell in love and got married to a charming and handsome man who adores me as much as I love him. We traveled the world together and have two cats and a dog. After nearly 2 decades in Chicago we recently moved to Baltimore – in some large part to be close to Johns Hopkins, which has some great specialists in vEDS. It's a slower pace of life and we are really enjoying the quirkiness of our new city. I spent the first year assembling my new medical team and I would say that was the hardest part about moving. However, I'm feeling pretty confident living so close to Johns Hopkins and I wake up happy every day.

> *"I don't want to see Daddy." I cried as I opened the door and jumped out of that car. Kristi Posival*

How did overcoming that challenge change how you perceived your health?

Once you realize your own strength in some capacity, it keeps things smaller. Well, my health is just that. My health. It's a small part of the whole. I think it's a bigger piece than most people but it can't define me. It can only be part of me.

What have you done to overcome low points throughout your journey?

Over the years I have tried lots of things to get through tough times. I have talked with therapists, psychiatrists, friends, family and anyone else who will listen in a deep and meaningful way. I have empathy for what others are going through because I understand life is complicated. I take comfort in knowing we all have a story and this one is mine. I have tried meditation and failed miserably. During low times my mind is in a panic so slowing it down is difficult. I would like to get better at it. There is something that I love to do and it helps release some tough emotions. Every three to four weeks I watch a terribly sad movie and sob. Many of the frustrations, fear, anger, sadness and other emotions created by EDS are very difficult to process. Stress is also terrible for EDS so I let my mind rest, start a good movie and let all my clogged up emotions out through tears. It's a simple cleansing that enables me to get a lot of stuff out. It's kind of like meditation I guess. If you're interested in trying it and need a movie suggestion, there is a documentary currently on Netflix called "Dear Zachary." It's so well done and just gut-wrenching in the most unimaginable ways.

I'm also annoyingly optimistic and a realist. I know vEDS will most likely cause my death one day, but today, right now, life is good. So I just go with that. When all that fails I like a glass of wine, or a toke of pot.

If you could offer one piece of advice to someone reading this book that felt disheartened by his or her diagnosis or health, what would you say?

Give yourself a break. You're trying the best you can. Offer that same break to others and trust they are trying the best they can. This diagnosis is a big label that means a whole lot of things. Take it in slowly. You're still you. You get to define the life you live.

Is there anything else that you would like to add that isn't covered in the answers above?

Challenge your doctors and yourself whenever you can. Ask many questions. Chances are you know a lot about your condition, your limitations and your strengths. For example, if your doctor says never lift more than 5 pounds, remind them your cat weighs 8 pounds and you can lift him without issue. I learned after many decades, avoiding physical exertion results in little or no strength, and that it is more harmful than a conservative approach to weights lifting that creates a little strength. If they say take 3000 mg of vitamin C everyday ask about a special diet in addition to that. Or a referral to a nutritionist. Anywhere in your life you can challenge yourself and your doctors for more knowledge leads to some good places.

It's very difficult to find a primary care physician with knowledge of EDS to treat your daily needs. Instead, find a doctor who has a curiosity that won't quit and one who wants to actively engage in discussions about you and your healthcare needs.

Last, the picture on back cover is one of my paintings. "Blue Girl" was painted in 2012, 6 years after my hand injury. It expresses the fear and isolation I often feel but try to quickly push out of my mind. It sold recently to a family who has a son with vascular EDS. For more images of my work visit www.KristiPosival.com.

WRITTEN BY KRISTI POSIVAL

Born in Green Bay, WI, Posival experienced tragedy at a young age. Her father, an engineer and painter, died suddenly at the age of 31 and was diagnosed with a rare genetic disorder during his autopsy. Posival was soon diagnosed with the same condition, Vascular Ehlers-Danlos Syndrome. Her formative years were tumultuous and painful. Doctors warned against any physical activity. An only child, Posival often found comfort with her paints and crayons, along with building forts with her imaginary friends. This marked the early stages of her fascination with figure drawing and exploring emotions through creative means.

In 1996, Posival graduated from Saint Norbert College with a BA in Graphic Communication and an emphasis in fine art. She immediately headed to Chicago. First priority, health care. Posival took a job in sales and design at a bar code company. A few years later she landed a great job as a graphic designer with a startup consulting firm trying to make corporate America a better place.

In 2002, Kristi left to pursue her passion of painting. From 2010 to present Kristi has had two solo shows and participated in several group shows. After moving from Chicago to Baltimore in 2014, she looks forward to getting her work shown on the east coast.

The purpose of art is washing the dust of daily life off our souls. – Pablo Picasso

For the Love of Pilates

I've always been athletic. I love physical activity and I started training to become a Pilate's instructor when I was 18. I ended up not finishing my training at that time because I was in college and it was too much for me to finish my schooling and train to be an instructor. After I graduated and had been working for a few years, I decided to do what I love which is Pilates and yoga. That's what I've been doing full time for about 7-8 years until about a couple of years ago when my pain started to become out of control. I began learning about EDS and my other major issues going on – spondylosis, spinal stenosis, severe sciatica pain, facet joint arthritis and facet joint cysts to name a few – that initially brought me to see my doctor.

EVERY SINGLE one of my doctors have said the only reason that I've made it so long without seeking medical intervention was because I kept myself in (pretty) great shape and kept my weight low and all the balance/stability training that goes along with Pilates and yoga that I've been doing since I was a teenager.

To enjoy the glow of good health, you must exercise.
– Sasha Cohen

I'm SO happy that my doctors all recognize that the main reason I have maintained a pretty dang good quality of life (until recently at least) was because of my physical activity. And they've all said it will be even more important to maintain my strength and level of activity moving forward into the future. I'm 36 (almost 37). Even though my activity level is really low right now because of my low back issues, I'm still doing what I can even if it's 25 minutes some days because to me, 25 minutes is better than 0 minutes!

So stay active and do what you can because it DOES make a difference and we will be far better off the more we can maintain or build muscle mass and stay active!!

WRITTEN BY MARY BOND

Watching My Mom

In 2012, our world changed. What was once normal became abnormal. There were suddenly fewer trips to the park, less time spent playing, and more of my time was spent trying to simply survive the insurmountable pain that ravaged my body. The following account is from my oldest son. The thoughts, emotions, and perception are all his own. –Mysti Reutlinger

My mom was hurting a lot. She spent all of her time in bed. I felt like I needed to help her. I wanted to make sure she had food to eat and something to drink. I also felt like I needed to take care of my younger brother. I made sure he ate and had something to drink. I kept him company and played with him while my mom was lying down.

There were times I wanted to give my mom a hug, but she said no because she hurt. When my mom did give me hugs, I could tell that it hurt her. Sometimes she got grumpy. I tried not to sit next to her so I wouldn't bump her and make her hurt more. I would sit on the floor next to her feet when she was on the couch.

My mom would make sure we could still go to church. She would make a smoothie to take with her and she had to take pain medicine. We had to come straight home after church because her pain would get worse again. I was happy to go to church and thanked her often.

My mom would see the doctor to get help for her pain. The medicine she took made her feel worse. So she decided to change her diet and stopped eating meat. We ate many salads and more fruits and vegetables. My mom started to get a little better.

When my mom was feeling better, she started exercising. She got even better with healthy foods and exercise. Feeling better meant we could do more things like going to the park, she went to more of my school events, and we traveled out of town to visit family and have fun.

There was one day when we went to Ft. Collins, Colorado to see a movie. My mom had the date wrong and we were a month early. Instead of going home, my mom took us out to eat. While we were eating, we decided to find something fun. My mom looked on her phone and found an arcade with putt-putt golf, laser tag, and go-carts. We ran around and played there and laughed a lot! We had cotton candy, too. That was the first time we traveled out of town just for fun since before my mom hurt so much.

There are still times when my mom hurts, but we are able to make the best of each day. We don't look at what we can't do, we focus on what we can do together.

Life is a series of experiences, each one of which makes us bigger, even though sometimes it is hard to realize this. For the world was built to develop character, and we must learn that the setbacks and grieves which we endure help us in our marching onward. – Henry Ford

AS TOLD BY JAY

Jay, also known as MC DarkMage, is 10 years old and lives with EDS. His hobbies include Minecraft, music, and art. He shares his passion for Minecraft at **MCDarkMage.com**

Artwork included with this story was created by Jay.

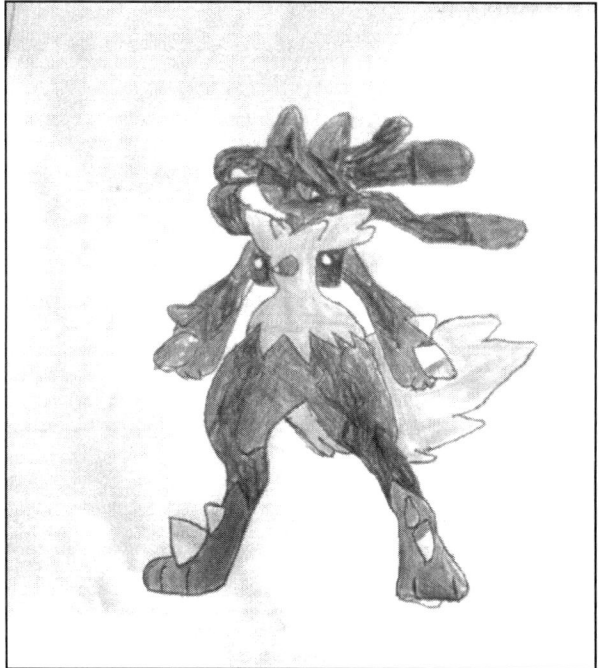

Couldn't Wouldn't Shouldn't

In 2004-2005, I began having severe pain in one arm, then both arms, and then both legs. With the pain came paralysis. I couldn't walk, I could barely talk, and I couldn't even dress myself. The ER doctors were stumped. I eventually regained my strength but occasionally the pain and bouts of paralysis will return with no warning and no triggers. It is terrifying. The idea I could wake up and be unable to function at all haunts me almost daily.

Does this mean I live in a hole and never come out? Absolutely not. It does mean I accomplish as much as I can on the days I am strong, so that I do not struggle as much when a bad day comes – and they do come.

My constant struggle with unbearable pain and strains seldom bothers me. I mean, come on, my mom and grandma had constant pain and made it – so could I. I am an overcomer. It wasn't until a few years ago I realized exactly how stubborn I am.

After my daughter was diagnosed and became progressively worse I began doing research on this unknown disease. Then she suffered more setbacks and was diagnosed with additional rare, often comorbid, health issues. I began researching deeper. I was disappointed that my searches left me frustrated and lost, feeling as though there was absolutely no hope for us, no support groups, no day-to-day life or suggestions.

Ever heard the phrase, "Mess with me and I will let it go. Mess with my kids and you will see a new kind of crazy?" EDS made the mistake of messing with my baby and I did go crazy. After my youngest managed to break an ankle and dislocate a shoulder while confined to a wheelchair, I decided it was time to quit working and homeschool her to see if she would improve. I pulled her out of school, set up a homeschooling program, and began asking the hard questions:

- Why was she so weak?
- Why was she worn out?
- Why was she so pale?
- *Why? Why? Why?*

These were all things I struggled with but didn't bother to research until they bothered my babies.

While this was taking place, my own health became worse. I suffered a life threatening miscarriage and my body took forever to recover as I could not stomach iron to replace the lost blood. I never stopped living my life through it all. I found ways to function and I even helped others, though I didn't realize it at the time.

Without a second thought, I developed ways to compensate for my constant pain, subluxations, and injuries. I would organize my schedule, home, and office to work for me. I knew reaching in a lower cabinet caused severe pain, so I found places for the most-used items within reach. If I was unable to pour something from a specific container due to weight, I would transfer it to a more accommodating container. I despised being unable to take care of my family! It wasn't until others began asking how I could live with the stress of my and my children's health issues did I realize the impact of these minor changes. I simply refused to let EDS ruin my life.

Is everyday perfect? No.
Do I accomplish all the things I want to? No.
Does EDS win? Sometimes, yes.
Will it run my life? No.

Does it make me depressed on occasion? Absolutely, but I shake off the dust and choose to accomplish what I can on any given day.

Some of my greatest challenges in living with EDS are the pain my girls experience, not always being able to commit to activities we want to do, and the frustration of feeling letdown. I make a "backup plan" every day, create standing and sitting to-do lists, blog, and find ways to be productive from my sofa or recliner – like researching, encouraging others, and finding solutions to what issues I face in the moment.

The day my youngest daughter was diagnosed with hypermobility EDS, I felt relief. Yes, relief. We **finally** had answers and I didn't have to feel like I was crazy anymore. After thirty plus years of questioning my own pain, it became accepted. Diagnosis didn't change my life, it simply provided me with a "named" enemy; something I could define – and fight.

I might not be able to do the things I want in a way I'm accustomed to doing them, but that doesn't mean I can't do them in a new way or replace the tasks with something else. Life is a choice and living is up to me. I may have EDS, but it doesn't have me.

A wise person always said, "Can't died in a cornfield along with couldn't, wouldn't, and shouldn't." Do you know why they died? Because they never tried. Instead of saying, "I can't do this!" How about asking, "What can I do?"

WRITTEN BY TINA MILLER

Tina is the mother of 3, wife of one and crazy owner of 4 cats and one dog. She spends her time looking after her children, operating two blogs, crafting and spreading awareness for EDS. She enjoys family, friends, craft and keeping a home.

Follow her blog at **TheZippyZebra.com**

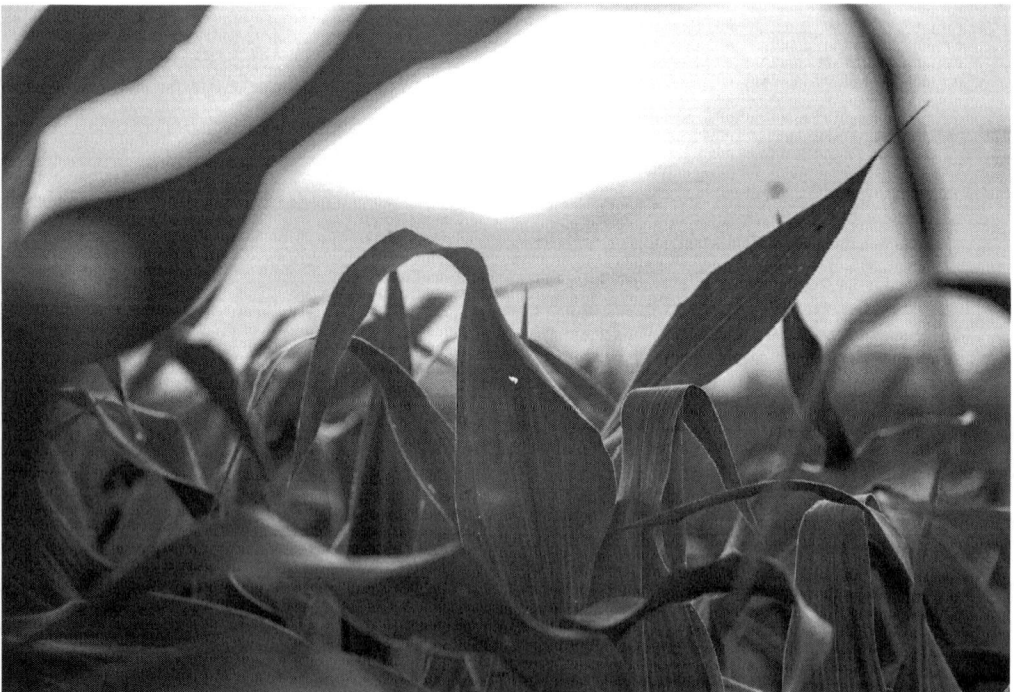

From Suffering to Living

Most of my adult life I'd been a control freak. I was an underachieving teenager, but grew to be a serious college student, a dedicated employee, and a woman with a reputation for achieving exactly what she wanted. In just a few years' time, I had already risen to honor roll, graduated from a respected private university, and begun a program that promised to end with a much sought-after specialty certification.

This sounds like a foolproof plan for a great life, right? Like every part of my life would just fall into place like the pieces of a giant puzzle? I believed that I could achieve every one of the goals I'd set for myself; after all, they weren't unreasonable goals. I worked diligently to ensure that my dreams became reality until an invisible illness emerged and turned my world around. From even the first day that Ehlers-Danlos Syndrome showed itself in my life, it began stealing my goals one at a time, until I found myself staring at a life I no longer recognized, filling with things I didn't want.

I'd never been what anyone would call the picture of perfect health, but I had always led a full, busy life with the help of antihistamines. I'd never broken a bone, needed a cast, or even had stitches; but by the time I reached my thirties, EDS had brought me the kinds of problems that aren't expected to happen to anyone until much, much later in life. The hallmark of my type of EDS, hypermobility, is a genetic defect that allows collagen to break down abnormally – leaving me with unstable joints, torn ligaments, and a pervasive arthritis that has affected most of my joints including my spine. This condition is not just extremely painful, but in my case, it was also a huge factor in my decision to leave the veterinary field. On some level, I suspect that my joint issues were probably inevitable, but to be perfectly honest, though I loved my work, the physical nature of my job probably didn't do much to stave off my abrupt exit. Having an extremely high threshold for pain allowed me to work through months when the pain was occasional and only mild, which, as it turned out, was still a lot longer than my doctor preferred. I worked full-time in spite of escalating pain for quite a while. I really felt like I was making the right decision for myself, both financially and medically. I carried on for months in the same state when, one evening, the pain suddenly became intolerable and I felt like I'd been hit by lightning from above. That was the day my stubbornness was put to bed and my doctor insisted that my veterinary career had to end if I wanted to maintain the ability to walk on my own.

I wasn't happy about leaving my career at all; I was downright beside myself, actually. For over a decade, my life had revolved around my job and where I wanted to take it, but in an instant, it was gone. There were no negotiations, no second chances, and no wait-and-see attitudes. He was clear, stop or expect severe, life-changing consequences. I left the doctor's office that day feeling a mix of emotions over my life no longer being within my control. I don't remember the details of the rest of that day, except that I cried, a lot. My husband, left feeling helpless and unable to say anything to make me feel better, assured me we'd get through this new obstacle together, whatever it would bring.

The first few weeks away from my job, I held onto the belief that one day, someday, maybe I'd be back to it once again. I had healed once, actually more like three or four times, and maybe I would get through this one too? As more time passed, it became apparent that I wasn't going to heal like I had before. I went to bed every night and awoke the next day with the same searing pain that moved through my joints in ways that only EDS can. Before that injury, I had always tried to avoid pain medications, but that kind of misery just wasn't manageable with an NSAID and an ice pack. I knew my body meant business this time. I couldn't even wash my own hair months after my last injury. I knew that even if I hated it, I'd have to accept that the chances of my being able to restrain a large, wiggling dog or an angry feline ever again, were fading with every passing day. The thoughts of going back to my job would have to change. Even if I could go back the veterinary field, I would never be able to do the same work I'd loved so much.

It took a long time for my body to even begin to recover from that injury. What my husband and I thought would be a few months slowly became years. The injuries have lessened, though they have never gone away. I'm the only person I know who can be injured walking on a level surface or reaching for a light switch – this is the life of a Zebra.

It was an enormous change to accept that my career was over for good. When I worked, fifty or sometimes sixty hours of my week would be filled with adrenaline and emergency shifts. I now had a million minutes in my weeks with nothing to do and no place in particular that I needed to be. Sure, I had medical appointments and pharmacy trips, often quite a number of them, but outside of those trips, I had the one thing I'd never had before: time and a whole lot of it. I'd started working as a young teenager and held a steady job (or two) since. Not once in my life was I ever able to wake up and have nothing to do. It felt weird and unnatural. Honestly, days when I had appointments and long drives to specialists felt more normal to me because they were tightly scheduled and often bordered on chaotic, exactly as my emergency shifts felt.

It was on the silent, quiet days that I struggled. I'd been busy for decades of my life and now, I just wasn't. I felt as if I had to start my life all over again and rediscover so many things about myself I just didn't know. What books did I want to read? Or would I rather write my own? Did I still enjoy sketching although it had been years since I had drawn a thing? Could I still identify the birds I'd watched in my carefree days as a child? Did I inherit my grandmother's affinity for baking? Could I cook without a microwave? I truly had no idea who I was anymore and it was overwhelming to now have every minute of every day to figure it out.

My last day on the job and the day I was given the official diagnosis were two of the hardest days of my entire life, but the days since have been some of the best. I took all that terrifying spare time and I turned it into something enjoyable, often even productive enough that my brain still appreciates the workout. Rather than live in denial, angry that the degree I earned could never be used for the purpose I had intended, I began to use it to write about more than just the life I had left behind. I was finally able to fully open my eyes to the possibilities that lie ahead of me, not just dwell on the disappointments. I had always loved to write, but had spent half of my life too busy to write on anything that wasn't a medical chart.

I knew if I ever really wanted to be happy again that I had to change the expectations I placed on myself and learn not to keep trying to live the life I once had. I needed to appreciate the life I had been given, even if I didn't ask for it. I knew I couldn't maintain the same pace that my much healthier-self had kept – to do so would risk reversing every bit of progress I'd made. I had been busy, far too busy by all reasonable standards, and I knew it. I seemed to believe that not moving a million miles an hour would make me a failure or somehow not as good as I could have been. When I finally accepted that pieces of my life had to change, I saw just how wrong I had been. It was the process of slowing down and accepting the changes I knew I had to make where healing, both physically and emotionally, came to pass. The hours I once filled with overnight shifts and rowdy animals were traded for mornings enjoying exceptional cups of coffee, walks on the beach with my husband, good books, and beautiful birds.

These days I walk through my life and I notice the small things I once overlooked that make my life amazing. I've come to love the way the perfect pen feels as it glides across the page, the sound of brilliant conversation, and the feel of a sunbeam on my face. I can unroll a blanket on the beach and enjoy an afternoon with my husband, doing very little of anything, and no longer find myself consumed by thoughts of what I probably should be doing instead. Being forced to change my whole life wasn't at all what I wanted or the future I had envisioned for myself. Life today isn't perfect by a long shot. I still have great days followed by really lousy days with painful joints and annoying migraines, but I no longer allow those hard days to hold me down. I've learned that there is an enormous difference between suffering from and living with EDS. Though I may never have the future I'd once envisioned or be exactly the woman I once was, I still enjoy a great life, full of the kind of happiness I'd once only managed to chase.

WRITTEN BY GWYNNE MOORE

I am a writer, editor, artist, wife, parent, and manic crocheter living with, and not suffering from, Ehlers-Danlos Syndrome. When I'm not reading a book or writing something of my own, I'm either on the beach, tangled up in yarn, or the reason our house always smells like fresh bread.

Multiple photos included in this anthology were captured by Gwynne Moore.

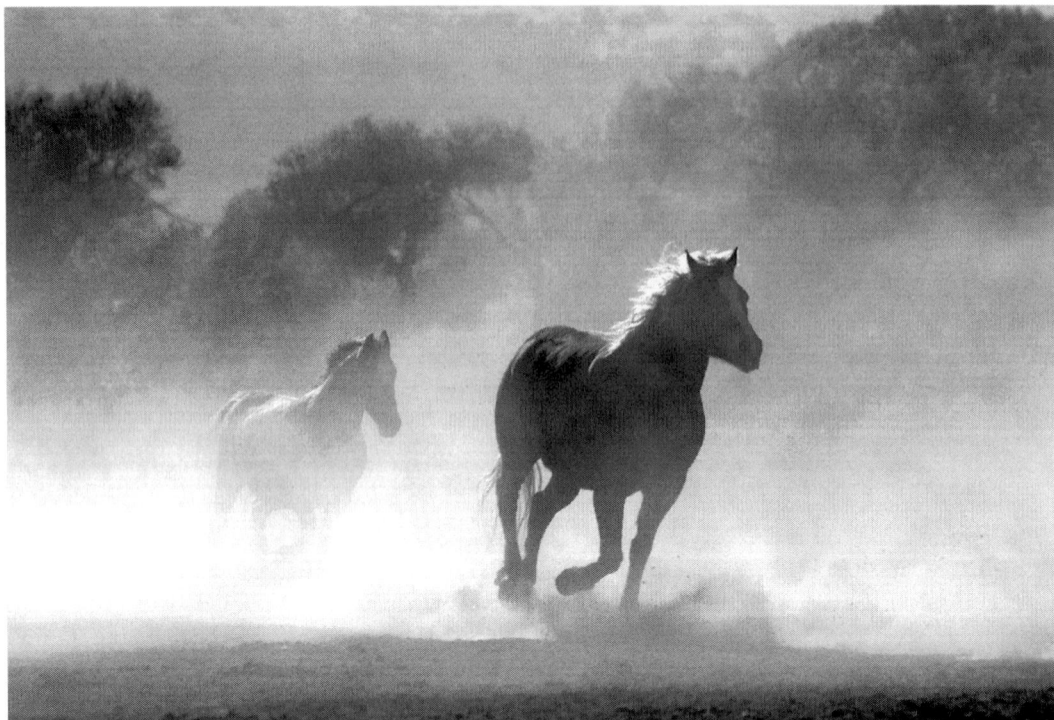

Adversity is the diamond dust Heaven polishes its jewels with. - Thomas Carlyle

Sometimes I Yell and Scream

The following is as-told-to Mysti Reutlinger by her youngest son with added commentary about his health and physical condition reflecting his perspective of living with Ehlers-Danlos Syndrome. Comments added by Mysti are italicized.

Can you tell me about your pain?

I have pain in my back and my legs. Sometimes my shoulders and arms hurt, too. My stomach hurts when I haven't gone to the bathroom for a while. I don't like when I feel pain.

What makes your pain feel better?

The massager (*tens unit*), warms baths, sometimes medicine helps, and walking helps my back, but gives me more pain in my feet. Bouncing around and not sitting in one place helps me, too.

Riding my bike helps me feel better. Exercises hurt when I'm doing them, but I feel much better after.

> *Balance/stabilization exercise routine aimed at teaching my children where their joints belong in space.*

Are there any things that make you feel worse?

Sitting in the car is really painful. I like to sleep because my back hurts.

Do you have trouble seeing?

In my left eye, I do. It makes me really angry if I can't see out of my right eye. I get hurt a lot when I wear an eye patch. That makes me scared.

> *Simon has high myopia consistent with Ehlers-Danlos Syndrome following Retinopathy of Prematurity that required laser treatment as an infant to prevent his retina from detaching. He has gone through patching for multiple years, but has become more apprehensive to the process, resulting in high anxiety, fear, and anger.*

What are some things you do that make writing and reading easier?

Sometimes writing with a pen is easier for me to see. I like when [my mom] writes words on the dry erase board because they are easier to read.

We utilize high-contrast tools to help Simon recognize his letters and numbers. He is beginning to read. He becomes extremely angry when reading from books if the font is too small. This has made an impact in his confidence in school. We are diligently encouraging him to rely upon the skills he has gained as well as venturing into learning braille by third grade to ensure he will be able to keep up with his peers in school.

Are there skills that you are learning at home or in school that will help you stay active?

My mom has taught me about what foods are really good for my body and which ones are bad. I try to eat more good food than bad. We go for walks and exercise, too. I also am learning about keeping my back straight.

What happens when you don't feel good? How do you react?

Sometimes I yell and scream. I get grumpy. Sometimes I hit my brother or my parents, too. I don't like the pain.

If a little boy or little girl were diagnosed with Ehlers-Danlos Syndrome, what would you tell them?

Everyone should be proud of who they are. If you don't feel good, let a parent know that you don't and see if a walk will help. If it doesn't, you might need some medicine or a massage.

AS TOLD BY SIMON

Simon is 6 years living with EDS. His hobbies include drawing, painting, and being an all-around active boy.

LOOKING UP

Man cannot aspire if he looked down; if he rise, he must look up.– Samuel Smiles

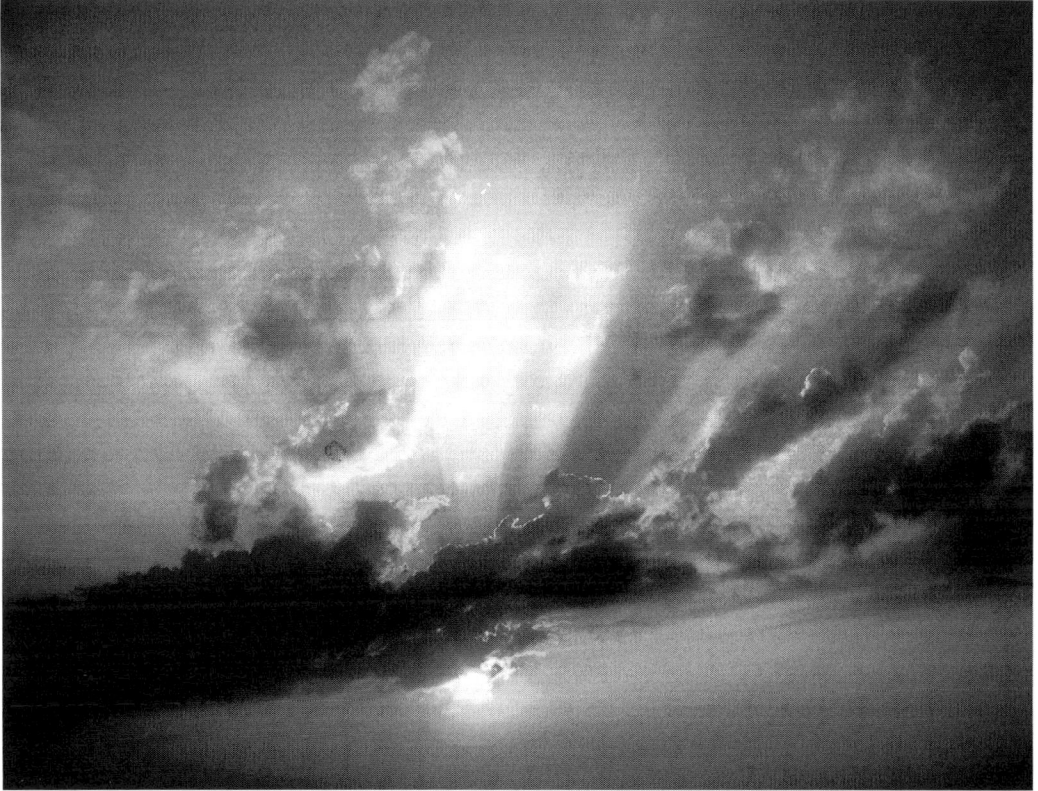

Certainly Uncertain?

The fields were covered with snow and the roads with ice. I have always been nervous of being too late, so it was no wonder I took the earliest bus possible to reach the hospital. As I was a couple of hours early I was surfing on my tablet to pass the time. I grew more and more nervous as I was waiting for my turn with the doctor and tried to calm myself. I was afraid of what my future would hold.

Would I be able to work? Would I be able to live with this pain? Would it ever get easier?

I decided to try to cheer myself up with some pictures of kittens. As I was swiping through all the cuteness, a notification popped up on the screen: unread mail. I opened up the application and the first thing I saw was a big red flag. **This was an important message.**

I read the subject and momentarily stopped breathing. It was regarding my application for a master's course. This was it, a final answer. I didn't dare open it at once. I looked around in the waiting room, feeling myself turning red. I had to get some privacy, so I went to the restroom. I was shaking so hard it took multiple tries to open it. My heart was beating so rapidly I thought it would jump out of my chest and run straight to the cardiac ward.

I couldn't believe it. The words of the e-mail started to make sense to me. It felt like I was still asleep on the morning bus. I stumbled out of the stall and went outside in the snow. My cheeks were burning and the cold did nothing. I called my mum hysterically, I couldn't control my feelings.

I was accepted!

My body and I don't see limb to limb, but this was my chance to form my future. I would fight with all my might for this to happen and enjoy every second possible.

WRITTEN BY VIKTORIA KESSLER

Zebra from Norway, studying Visual Communication in Cheltenham, England. Multimedia artist with a passion for books. Learn more at viktoriakessler.com

From Dream Job to Paralysis

In 2006, at age 20, I suffered bilateral partial lower limb paralysis due to an EDS injury caused in part by an inexperienced therapist. For 9 months, I had no sensation when someone touched my legs and I couldn't actually feel my legs underneath me. I had some minor urinary involvement but thankfully I was still, for the majority anyway, able to control my bladder and bowels.

The major turning point when this crisis occurred was after about 2 weeks. I was lying in a hospital bed (where I ultimately spent a month before being sent home to rehabilitate) and had been told about a week earlier that they didn't know when or even IF I would get feeling/sensation back in my legs and that I needed to prepare for the possibility that I might not get them back. If I did, sensation would likely be altered. For the following week, I will admit, I wallowed… I screamed and cried, moaned and muttered. Stating "It's not fair" and asking "Why me?" because there I was, in the absolute high point of my life with an amazing job offer, a large group of friends, an amazingly supportive (and patient!) family…and I was in hospital, paralyzed, not knowing if I'd ever walk again.

In that second week I pulled on my big girl panties and demanded to know how best improve my chances of regaining feeling, sensation and the ability to walk back…and that was physiotherapy – LOTS of it too! I worked hard at it because I was determined to regain SOME control back over my legs AND my life. While in hospital, I decided I was going to continue my studies and signed up for full time correspondence course. I figured I would have some free time in my foreseeable future and I was determined that once I could walk again, I would work again. So for 9 months I did hours of physiotherapy a day and then hours of study, alternating them until my body hurt and my eyes became fatigued…but it all paid off. While I never regained the same strength or sensation I had had previously, I learned to walk again with the help of my parents, a massage therapist, physiotherapy, manual movement and good old-fashioned determination. **I learned to walk again!**

Prior to that injury and subsequent paralysis, I had considered myself indestructible. My health was a nuisance with regular injuries, pain, fatigue, and all the other issues that come along with EDS. I thought if I convinced myself I was unbreakable, I would BE unbreakable, and so when the injury and paralysis occurred, I felt weak. I believed I wasn't trying hard enough to be unbreakable. Because I never regained full strength or feeling back in my legs, and the general overall deterioration of my health over the last 10 years, I still feel like I am weak at times. But, at the same time, I also look back and see what my body managed to overcome and think "Wow…I did that…while my body was badly broken for a time, I still managed to overcome that." These days, while my health is a definite hindrance to my life, and my body deteriorating much faster than I would like or had even expected, I feel I am a stronger person mentally for it all, that I can try to meet any challenge my health throws at me head on, and that I CAN triumph over it. This doesn't mean I don't have difficult moments like the reflection in this poem:

The Face

The face hides more pain than you can realize...
The smile covers the words that want to come out...
The eyes hide the tears that have yet to be shed...
The mind betrays all that you see…
It's all a show…
A show for which I pay the price…
Just so you don't know…
How wounded I truly am…
Alone with my pain…
Swallowed whole by agony…
I cry the unshed tears…
But there's always more to come…
Clawing my way back to sanity…
Forever teetering on the brink…
Making sure the face is set…
Making sure it doesn't crack…
I do this to spare you…
You can't ever understand my pain…
Just acknowledge and accept it…
That this is just my way…
Broken on the inside…
Desperate, angry and hurt…
No chance to cope or to fall apart…
The world beckons me away…

I find it hard to sit around and do nothing while I recover… it is when I do nothing that I start to get REALLY depressed. I feel like EDS and all the comorbidities have taken everything from me. So, while yes, I need a psychologist sometimes to talk over my thoughts and feelings and to help acknowledge and to deal with them in a safe and productive manner, I like to be proactive.

I have done a number of rounds of cognitive behavior therapy, partaken in meditative therapies and art therapy, and most recently, a pain management course offered by one of the universities here. I find that if I can understand something, I can overcome it, so for me, knowledge IS power... the power to overcome each challenge in the present and move forward with my beautifully broken life.

WRITTEN BY KYLIE LANG

I am soon to be 30 years old and have many medical diagnoses', the most life-affecting of which are EDS, fibromyalgia, dysautonomia, endometriosis and adenomyosis. I have a wonderfully caring and supportive fiancé, a dog called Snoopy and two cats called Juju and Caesar.

No one saves us but ourselves. No one can and no one may. We ourselves must walk the path. - Buddha

Appearances are Deceptive

People with EDS know that appearances are deceptive.

I was born in the northern industrial town of St. Helens, England on the first of June 1950 at a quarter past two; precisely one half hour after my brother, Victor. My early years were spent in a simple two up, two down terraced house that had a toilet at the bottom of the yard. By the time I'd progressed to grammar school we'd moved to a very nice house in a posher part of town; so posh in fact that it had an inside toilet.

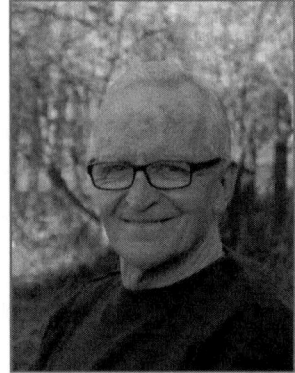

I left school in 1969 and worked in the Health Service for ten years before becoming a teacher, a career that lasted until my retirement in 2009. I got married in 1973 and subsequently produced three children who have provided me with soon-to-be fifteen beautiful grandchildren. For all intents and purposes I have lived a very ordinary, conventional life. At sixty-four years of age I look reasonably fit. I am retired. I sing with Hull Male Voice Choir; I can limp round a golf course and I like gardening.

I have a problem however, one that has dogged me all my life. I am not ill, but I have suffered a multiplicity of injuries including cuts requiring 200 stitches; a broken femur; several broken bones; dislocated joints; ruptured knee ligaments and catastrophic bruising to my right shin (the bruise was bigger than my shin).

The first occurred when I was a baby. My father was playing with me in the front room. I crawled under a sideboard to gather a ball that had rolled past me. My parents immediately recognized that something was wrong as I began crying and did not come out from under the furniture. My father pulled me out feet first and to his horror, was greeted by my bloodied face. I had split my forehead from top to bottom in three different places. The white scars are still visible to this day. My parents checked the sideboard and found nothing untoward. I had apparently cut myself on nothing.

As a result I was referred to a consultant pediatrician who inaccurately diagnosed me as suffering from "unconfirmed haemophilia." My medical problem was so rare that they simply didn't know what was wrong with me. It was not until I was nineteen that I was finally diagnosed as having Ehlers-Danlos Syndrome.

As a result of this misdiagnosis, both my parents and I were not given the correct help and guidance until much damage had already been done to my body. Photographs of my childhood all share the same feature: Some part of my body is bandaged and in a sling or a plaster cast.

Despite this, the photographs show an apparently happy little boy squinting into the holiday sunshine. The pictures lie however. I was not happy. In fact I was very troubled, but no one knew it. I have suffered much emotional damage as a result of the physical injuries and have only now begun to come to terms with it. My doctor said I was just accident-prone. My friends said I was an accident waiting to happen. Everybody laughed at my apparent clumsiness. I laughed. It was my only defence. It wasn't funny. No one could help me and the harder I tried, the more problems I seemed to have. There were no support groups and even if there had been, there were no forms of communication like Facebook. Only now do I realise how isolated I have been. Even when they gave me a correct diagnosis, it didn't help. I was told that there were 87 recorded cases, which made me the 88th. What was the point in seeking help? No one knew what the hell I was talking about.

Things have got better over the years, but it was not until New Year's Day 2008, that a real change began. I fell off a ladder in my garage and broke my femur. I was laid up for more than 6 months. During that time I found myself asking, "If I had died what would I have been most unhappy about?" The answer was that I would have been annoyed that I hadn't completed the book I was trying to write.

Braver Than All The Rest draws on my experiences as a Special Needs co-ordinator in a Sixth Form college. As I wrote the novel about others' problems I realised that I had a story of my own to tell. My second book is my autobiography "An Accident Waiting To Happen." Writing helped me come to terms with who I am. I couldn't be a rugby player or a footballer. I tried, but spent more time in hospital than on the pitch, but I found I could write. It took 60 years to find happiness, but now it's here. I am at peace with myself. Life is worth living if you can find a way to enjoy it.

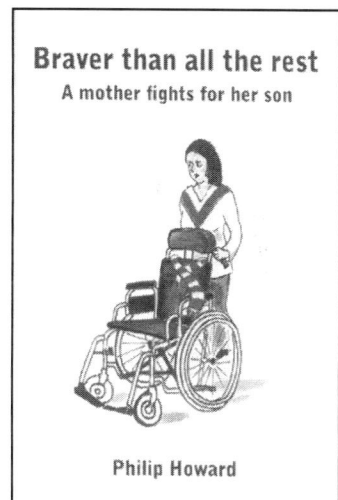

Braver than all the rest
A mother fights for her son

Philip Howard

WRITTEN BY PHILIP HOWARD

Phillip Howard is the author of *Braver Than All The Rest* and *An Accident Waiting To Happen*. You can find him on Twitter @imphilhoward

About Braver Than All The Rest: Dave and Sarah Burgess are devastated when their young son Karl is found to have muscular dystrophy. Then another tragedy hits the family hard. But the family are committed to do the best they can for Karl, who has a passion for rugby league. Based in Castleton, a Yorkshire town near the border with Lancashire, Karl's determination to get the most out of life, despite his disability, inspires those around him, in particular Chris Anderton, one of the Castleton Rugby League Club players, who is coming to the end of his career in the game. A moving novel of family life and rugby league.

Published in 2010 at £9.95, special offer £9.00 direct from London League Publications Ltd. Credit card orders via www.llpshop.co.uk , orders by cheque to LLP, PO Box 65784, London NW2 9NS

The doctors said I had
unconfirmed haemophilia.

People said I was clumsy, a clown,
an accident waiting to happen.

They were wrong!

200 stitches; a broken femur;
broken bones in my feet;
3 sprained ankles;
dislocated kneecaps;
ruptured knee ligaments;
a broken scaphoid;
traumatic bruising to my shin
and a dislocated shoulder.

These were the gifts that
Ehlers Danlos syndrome
had bestowed upon me. I had always fought back and
recovered but at fifty eight years of age I had had enough.
I lay on the floor in my garage with the fallen ladder as
my companion, listening to the siren of an
approaching ambulance. I thought to myself
"I have to find a way to make all this stop. If I survive."

Philip Howard

AN ACCIDENT WAITING TO HAPPEN | PHILIP HOWARD

AN ACCIDENT WAITING TO HAPPEN

a life with Ehlers Danlos Syndrome

The Bubble

When I was eleven years old, I saw more doctors than I could count. I saw specialists of all sorts who were more blinded by their specialties than the experts that they proclaimed. For three years I searched for an answer. Three years of pain, confusion, frustration and mystery with the underlying cause of something that could be learned in three minutes.

Time after time, I would enter a doctor's office claiming a 9 out of 10 on the pain scale and see the shock of their faces when I would bend my body. "If you were in that much pain I'd be scraping you off the ceiling," said one. "Come see this girl's back!" screamed another to her colleague. What they did not realize at the time was that I do not belong in the circus like the girl pictured in their medical books. I, in fact, have Ehlers-Danlos Syndrome.

The funny thing about those doctors who couldn't tell me what was wrong was that they instead told me what I shouldn't be doing. I once had a knee that would not stop dislocating as I played soccer and saw a doctor who said, "hasn't anyone ever told you not to play sports?" as if the fourteen-year old me should know better, should have given up what she loved because of this no-named-mystery-illness. Devastated and dismayed, my physical therapist combated the rude remark by saying, "hey, it beats a bubble!" And so it began, my quest to live my life because it beats being confined by a bubble.

The obstacles that I face in an attempt to live my life vary anywhere from when I play sports to when I go to school to going to the pharmacy to pick up my prescriptions. Living with EDS isn't easy, being active while having EDS can be downright difficult at times, but it is never impossible. If I could go back ten years and tell eleven-year-old me one thing I would tell her, "don't let them stop you." If you let them stop you, then you would have never played collegiate sports. I would have never met the girls who became my sisters. I would never have become the leading goal scorer on both the soccer and lacrosse teams. I would have never received all-conference honors as a freshman. So what if I might be exhausted and in pain after a game, so what if I have to literally tape my joints together, so what if I may have only been able to play competitively for two years. "You did it," I would say, "and it was amazing."

The hardest part about living with an invisible illness is that people cannot tell that you are sick. I once had a woman in Starbucks publically yell at me for using my handicap placard, claiming I should save it for someone who was "actually handicapped." If only she had put on her x-ray glasses that morning and could see my hips dislocating, spine compressing and brain falling out of my skull, she might have understood why I was using it that day. But, in life, there will always be those people who tell you that you cannot do something. There will always be those doctors who have never heard of the disease, those people who can't tell that you are sick, or simply the people who are defeated by obstacles the size of an ant hill. No matter who it is, why would you let them stop you?

Living with Ehlers-Danlos brings more daily challenges than someone may expect. Careful, don't stand up too quickly, you might pass out. Did you check to make sure your ankles weren't dislocated before you hopped out of bed? Class, physical therapy, babysitting, AND grocery shopping? Not today. It is a balance and a struggle and the best thing that has ever happened to me. This thing that causes my body to fall apart, this thing called Ehlers-Danlos Syndrome, has taught me more than I could ever learn in a classroom. It has taught me more about myself than I ever thought possible and has made me the strong, resilient woman I am today.

I consider myself lucky because I have EDS. It has made me who I am today; it has shaped the person I want to become. Because of EDS I have a reason to fight. I have a reason to get up in the morning, to take on the world, to live my life, and beat the odds. I believe in things happening for a reason. I believe that I was placed on this earth with the debilitating disease so that I could show and share my strength with the people around me. Despite the tears I shed from the pain after a game, despite the challenges I have just to climb a flight of stairs, it is worth it. Despite the glares I get when I park in a handicap spot, despite the pity looks I get when I have my neck brace on, it is worth it. Despite the challenges I have to get out of bed every day, despite the memory issues I face in my classes to become a doctor, it is worth it. Despite the doctor's appointments, the needle sticks, and the surgeries, it is worth it. Despite the fears I have, the pain I dread, and the struggles I face, it is all worth it because one day I will be able to look back and say, "look what I did" because I lived a life that beat a bubble.

WRITTEN BY VICTORIA L. GRAHAM

Victoria Graham is a student at Eastern University pursuing a bachelor's degree in biology on the pre-medical track, with plans to go on to medical school and enter into the medical field. She has published biological research into the National Center for Biotechnology Information Database, and has worked as a research assistant and teaching assistant at Eastern University.

Diagnosed at age 13 with Ehlers-Danlos Syndrome, Victoria was a competitive gymnast and an avid competitor in both soccer and lacrosse. Not one to let anything keep her down, Victoria continued playing soccer and lacrosse through high school and into college, utilizing a menagerie of braces, tape, and prayers to hold her body together. Prior to her recent cranial and spinal surgeries that put a halt to sports, Victoria was the leading scorer for Eastern University's women's lacrosse and soccer teams.

In addition to Ehlers-Danlos Syndrome, Victoria also has dysautonomia, postural orthostatic tachycardia syndrome, mast cell activation disorder, Raynaud's syndrome, and hypokalemic periodic paralysis.

Victoria is passionate about philanthropy, especially in organizing events to support children with medical issues and families who are experiencing difficult challenges. Victoria resides in Maryland with her father, mother, and brother. She enjoys painting, baking, and watching the Food Network.

"In matters of truth and justice, there is no difference
between large and small problems, for issues
concerning the treatment of people are all the same."
– Albert Einstein

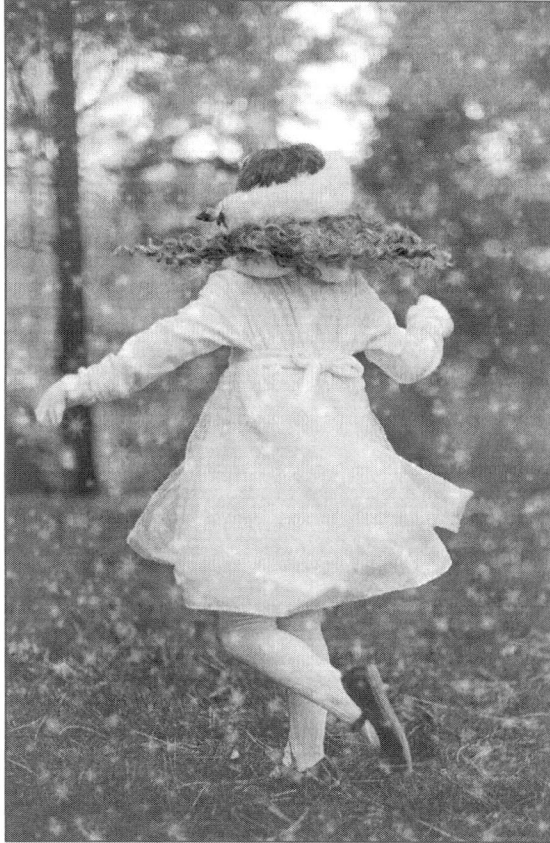

The Dance

I have danced around the room since I turned two,
Who would have imagined what I was able to do.
I touch my toes to my nose both front-ways and back,
Many thought that I would eventually crack.
I never thought my blessing could double as a curse,
My shoulders would come out of socket while reaching for my purse.
I live my life differently than I did before,
Never limiting myself by opening every door.
I may feel pain or my skin may look like lace,
You will never see it on my face.
I love my body with every ounce,
Even if my skin has a little extra bounce.
I am not affected just by my skin,
But every joint and muscle within.
Embrace who you are and never hate it,
Simply listen to your body and evaluate it.
It takes some trial and error to find your limits,
Once you do, simply live within it.

If I can do this, you can too!

WRITTEN BY REBECCA GILMAN

I lived with EDS for almost 25 years and it helped me pursue my dreams of being a dancer when I was younger and I never let it change how I have lived my life. Once I was officially diagnosed I have had to stop dancing, but it has never gotten me down. It is one aspect of my life that makes me who I am. It does not define me.

*I want to inspire people. I want someone to look at me
and say because of you, "I didn't give up!" - Unknown*

When All Else Fails, Join the Circus

As 2012 drew to a close, I hit a new low. After a year and a half of trying treatment after treatment for psoriatic arthritis, the effectiveness of my latest regimen was waning. To make matters worse, I had also been diagnosed with POTS the summer prior, and Ehlers-Danlos was the suspected cause. After having been on a very successful career path at a top consulting firm, I was now on disability, spending most of my time in bed, bound by the chains of severe chronic pain, dizziness, and fatigue. My rheumatologist had run out of options – it was time for me to come off my biologic medication and prepare to start IV infusions of Remicade – the biggest gun she had left in her arsenal.

Like many things in the life of a patient with a chronic debilitating disease, the prospect of switching medications proved more complicated than it would seem on the surface. Given the degree of immune suppression that was likely to ensue on the new medication, my doctor wrote me a prescription for a preemptive shingles vaccine. Despite having a prescription in hand, pharmacy after pharmacy turned me away, saying this would be considered "off label" administration due to my young age. Even after finding a pharmacist who was willing to give the vaccine, further delays ensued while awaiting the vaccine shipment to come in and allowing for my body to respond and make antibodies.

I was in incessant daily pain, and I was desperate. I decided I had to do something. As a physician, I had always looked to traditional Western medicine as my first line defense, but it seemed to be running out of options for me. In the intervening months, I tried a myriad of things – supplements, acupuncture, you name it. But there were two things I did that completely changed the course of my illness and my outlook on life.

On January 1, 2013, I made the decision to change to the Paleo diet. I intuitively knew the foods I was eating were not making me feel well. After hearing stories of others who had improvement in their autoimmune conditions after eliminating processed foods, I figured it was worth a try. The next day, I threw everything out of my pantry and fridge and completely started over. The first couple of trips to the grocery were multi-hour lessons in label-reading, but I quickly got the hang of which foods, brands, and flavors I should look for.

The following week, I made what was perhaps an even more game-changing decision – I started working out again 5 days a week. I had always been very active growing up, and before my illness set in, I was race walking 25 miles a week and working out with a personal trainer. All that had gone by the wayside when the pain in my hips and back and the effects of POTS became too severe. I knew I needed to get my body moving again, but the old ways of exercise weren't going to fly. I needed something a little less punishing to my joints, and it had to be so much fun that I would push past all of the pain and fatigue to do it.

I was fortunate at the time to belong to a gym that had a great selection of group fitness classes and a tremendously supportive community feel. My trainer suggested I try Zumba. I had danced for years growing up, and she knew I would enjoy it. That first class, I couldn't make it through more than one song in a row without having to sit down and rest, but it didn't matter…I was DANCING. It was pure joy!! Sure, I had to learn to dance in a knee brace and become a master at kinesio tape, but there was nothing that was going to keep me from going back for more. What started as Zumba expanded into spinning, water aerobics, TRX, Pilates, yoga, and other forms of group exercise. I learned that it was OK to not be able to do everything right away. If I had a new instructor, I would just tell them about my limitations, and they would work with me to modify accordingly. I was not bashful about sharing my story with my classmates, and they rallied around me to keep my spirits high.

In February of 2013, the diagnosis of hypermobile type Ehlers-Danlos Syndrome was confirmed, and I was told what I already suspected after those first six weeks…I was doing the right thing. My body needed to rebuild muscle tone to both stabilize my joints and control the symptoms of POTS. I could feel a difference already and nothing was going to stop me now. What started as one class a day, 5 days a week quickly grew to 12 hours a week. I scheduled the classes in advance and stuck to them as I would any other committed appointment. I didn't want to let my friends and my instructors down. Most importantly, I didn't want to let myself down. Sure, I would sometimes have a tough day and have to sit one out, but I would make the time up on another day. And, I built variety into my routine so as to minimize the stress on any particular joints or muscle groups by doing the same repetitive activities day after day.

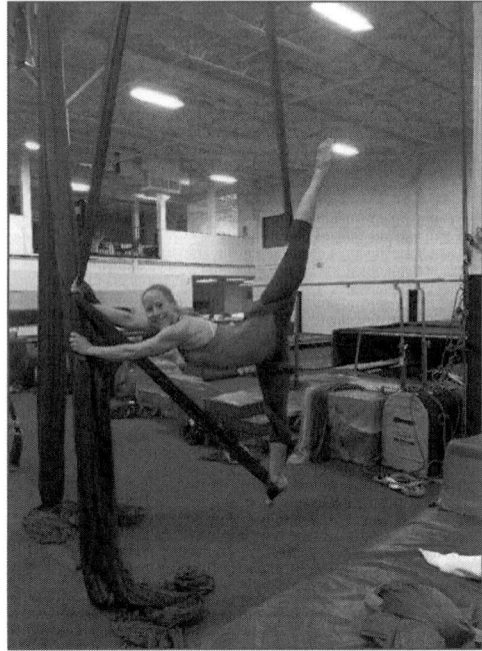

After three months, the improvement in my condition was remarkable. I was in less pain and had more energy than I had in years. Not only did I not have to start the IV infusions – I was off all biologics for a total 6 months until finally restarting self-injections after having my first flare. I began traveling and interviewing for jobs, and started back to work full time in June 2013.

My journey continues to evolve. I am now up to 15 hours a week of exercise and have become an avid circus arts aerialist and Pilates enthusiast. My core has stabilized to the point where back pain – which used to have me sleeping countless nights on the floor instead of in bed – is, most days, a minor nuisance. My physical strength and endurance now exceed that of most of the women with whom I train, many of which are half my age.

As does anyone with a chronic illness, I still have daily struggles. Joint subluxations and muscle spasms cause pain in a myriad of locations. I still take way more naps than I would like to, and I have to set an alarm a full hour before I actually want to get out of bed to take medications for POTS and narcolepsy, or I absolutely can't get going. Forget trying to actually go to the gym in the morning…that just lands me right back in bed! But, with some patience and creativity, a new job that better fits my needs yet still fulfills my passion, and a hearty dose of perseverance; I have found a routine that works for me.

My greatest lessons in this journey have been to be my own advocate, to surround myself with a network of supporters, to forgive my own imperfections, and to follow my passions. I hope you will join me.

WRITTEN BY CHRISTINE HALE

When you have the confidence, you can have a lot of fun. And when you have fun, you can do amazing things. - Joe Namath

Ehlers-Danlos Syndrome Isn't Rare

It's Just Rarely Diagnosed

Life is definitely what happens while we're busy making other plans. I knew at an early age that I was different somehow, but not quite sure how. I was smaller than most, easily picked on and into different things than most of the girls at school. I was also much bendier than most until my teens. But no one ever said anything about this being unusual. My parents were too busy managing their own issues and challenges and my older sister and I just got on with our lives as adult children of alcoholics as best we could after we graduated from high school.

I struggled to get along with the majority of girls and people my age, always seeking older friends and mentors. Then I started experiencing chronic lower back pain in my early twenties. I also battled some depression and anxiety that doctors loved to focus on instead of my increasing pain and physical troubles. I would have various odd issues (ganglion cysts, hemorrhoids, neuromas) and paradoxical reactions to various medications and procedures (anaphylaxis to bees and contrast dye, vomiting for days after minor surgeries, and allergic to many antibiotics). I also had severe environmental allergies to grass and tree pollens, cats and mold, practically wearing a Kleenex box all spring and summer. But again no one ever thought this was remarkable or urged me to make a note of it so I didn't, at least not on paper.

I struggled to get going with work out of college – I was plenty smart and loved taking direction but battled chronic fatigue and increasing pain and IBS in my 20s. Although I was ultimately diagnosed with chronic fatigue syndrome in Seattle at that time, the diagnosis never felt quite right to me, like there was a piece or pieces missing. I was one point shy of a fibromyalgia diagnosis so was left to suffer unsupported despite my ten very real tender points accordingly. I finally settled into some administrative work after moving back to Portland to help my aging and ailing father who was passing out from what I now recognize as likely POTS attacks in hindsight despite his drinking history. (He was too habitual to binge.)

We got my dad back on his feet and I got on with life, always wanting to write a book about my experience as an odd duck with an unidentified chronic pain and fatigue condition but never quite got around to it. (My first working title was "Gullible's Travels" but a smart travel writer beat me to it, darn it!) I worked a variety of jobs, bought a couple of houses and launched a database consulting career but not any writing. My pain and fatigue slowly steadily increased and I learned to just suck it up and carry on, as no one seemed interested in hearing about it, often one-upping me with their own experiences, or just dismissing me outright. (The story of my life as you can see.)

My first good clue to what was really wrong came after injuring my upper back while collating medical records in 2007. (I took T3-T5 out twisting not lifting.) Three different practitioners including my great PT and a chiropractor all independently called me "plastic" during my treatment, and the physical therapy made me worse until I gave it up and finally switched to acupuncture in desperation. (A great move in hindsight.) My massage therapist then suggested I might be "hypermobile" when I shared this experience with her, a word I'd never heard but which really fit when I googled it. But my doctor still didn't think I had anything worth pursuing so I once again carried on with life as best I could despite my issues.

Fast forward to early 2012 when I suddenly weakened severely from head to toe and went from walking to wheelchair in just three weeks for no apparent reason! I had not had any trauma or viral illness that often trigger fibromyalgia flares like this either. At the height of my onset "storm" (or "cascade" as some doctors prefer) my right leg subluxed along with my fingers, ribs and toes and I split my right sacroiliac (SI) joint leaving me literally "dragging a leg" and wheelchair bound for six months. I finally got to see a medical geneticist on Valentine's Day who diagnosed me at almost 45-years old with the hypermobile type of Ehlers-Danlos Syndrome (EDS) which clearly runs in my late dad's family if not also my late mother's in 20/20 hindsight. We ruled out some more rare types via blood tests also. I had to work from memory and piece together what family history I could from my remaining elderly aunts at the time. And I suddenly found and met "my people" in several great online support groups. Along with finding several common comorbidities including mast cell activation syndrome (a form of MCAD) and autism spectrum disorders among others, I finally had the answers I needed to write my book!

I'm eternally grateful for all of the incredibly helpful advice and recovery tips from my many fellow sufferers online by guiding me rebuild my shattered body. Although there is no cure, I have been thrilled to resume walking again, albeit with a crutch. A rigorous nutritional and physical therapy program includes high dose vitamin C plus several cofactors (calcium, magnesium and zinc among others) along with probiotics and an organic allergy-free whole foods diet. This has allowed me to ditch my pain pills again except for occasional break-through pain after busting too many moves.

While I might not win any foot races and can still paralyze from sitting too long in the wrong position, I'm twice the Jan I was three years ago and continue to slowly improve on the whole, trending upward like the stock market. I even managed to bike across the Golden Gate Bridge the summer of 2014! Of course I now dearly hope to share my best insights, tips and tricks with as many as possible to help others enjoy similar quality of life and recovery despite this painful condition, and shorten the road to diagnosis for my fellow long-suffering patients. As I've told my friends since 2012, my life isn't over, it's just different - and happy now that I have some answers finally!

WRITTEN BY JAN GROH

Ehlers-Danlos Syndrome survivor and blogger, Jan Groh has long wanted to share her painful 25+ year journey to a correct diagnosis, and now finally feels able. She is turning her talent for distilling complex information into digestible bits from the database field to the medical field and working on her first book: Oh! That's Why I'm So Tired! In it, she hopes to help shorten the diagnostic journey for others and save both patients and doctors needless suffering from misdiagnosis and misunderstanding around this poorly recognized and incredibly wide-ranging systemic condition.

See more of her writing and watch for her book at: **OhTwist.com**.

Education is the most powerful weapon which you can use to change the world. - Nelson Mandela

Police Wife with Rare Disease

Helps Organize History Making Rally in Support of Police Officers

WASHINGTON, DC- Rachel Bowman has worn many hats in her life. Like many women, she's been a wife and a mother, but that's where what is typical about her stops. She is now part of a trio of women responsible for putting together the End the Madness - Sea of Blue March and Rally set to take place from noon to 3 pm on Saturday, January 17, 2015 in Washington DC. The initial purpose of the event was to show support for local police officers like her husband, but over the last week their walk has grown into not just something global for their cause, but a major accomplishment for Rachel.

Like the other wives involved in this event, Rachel is also the wife of a police officer, but unlike her partners, she's a woman on another kind of mission, for good reasons too. Ms. Bowman is a stroke survivor with a complicated medical chart due to Ehlers-Danlos Syndrome and a woman with a defiant streak.

Rachel is still young by most standards, yet she has already endured more in the last decade and a half than most will ever experience in a lifetime. She has had brain and neck surgery, nerve damage arising from a minor stroke, followed by a number of additional surgeries including a second neck surgery to correct complications from the first. She has endured years of chronic pain, crippling migraines and years of partial bed rest as a result of Ehlers-Danlos Syndrome.

EDS is an inherited disorder caused by a defect in collagen that is still considered to be relatively rare by most medical professionals. So much so, those members of the EDS community have taken to referring to themselves as Zebras The name is a play on the phrase, "When you hear hoof beats look for horses, not zebras," meant to encourage medical professionals to rule out more common issues before considering unusual ones such as Ehlers-Danlos Syndrome. This zebra reference has come to symbolize the EDS community and why Rachel Bowman will be wearing a zebra-striped ribbon this Saturday.

Arriving at Ehlers-Danlos as a diagnosis is often a long, painful road filled with visits to a number of different specialty physicians, one Rachel knows too well. Much of the body is comprised of collagen, including the skin, blood vessels, muscles and ligaments. This disorder causes a myriad of unusual symptoms as well as extreme pain and joint instability or, in cases such as Rachel's, both. She can still recall a time not so long ago when simply getting out of bed was so tiring and taxing on her body that the idea of shopping by herself was nearly impossible, or planning a major event such as this one, would have been nearly impossible.

Her journey began over a decade and a half ago, then, for no apparent reason at all, Rachel suddenly began to notice changes in her overall health. It was during a time when she was nearly bedridden, having been told by doctors that her chances of ever living a normal life again were nearly impossible and that her current condition was likely to persist for the rest of her life, that Rachel's medical condition suddenly began to improve. The progress was slow at first, but by the end of 2014, she was not just out of bed, but once again engaged in her life for the first time in years.

Showing policemen like her husband that they are appreciated is one of Rachel's goals for Saturday's events, but, for her, there's more. "What I want from this march is for my message to be heard around the nation. Cops need to know that we appreciate and support them, but I also want to show other chronic illness patients, especially those with Ehlers-Danlos Syndrome, that no matter what illness you may have, however bad you may feel today, tomorrow can always be better." Ms. Bowman continues, "In your darkest hours, don't give in to despair, please don't give up. I have been there too, a lot of people have in fact, but I forged on and look at what I'm doing now! The fact that my doctors though I would never have any quality of life is important to me because I refused to listen. I refused to give up and I told them so! I want what I am doing right now with this rally to give others hope. There have been so many articles written lately about others with this disorder dying, I'd like to show what one of us can do when she wants it badly enough."

SUBMITTED BY RACHEL BOWMAN / WRITTEN BY GWYNNE L. MOORE

Q&A with Contessa Courtney

What type of EDS do you have and when were you diagnosed?

I am what we call a stiff Zebra, EDS Type 3 – not hypermobile. I have never had any joint hypermobility. I do have constant problems with muscle tightness, cramps, aches and pain.... but after reading about the problems others with EDS have, in a way I feel lucky not to have hypermobility, which causes many additional problems. I do have severely debilitating "fatigue" which prevents me from leading a normal life and confines me to bed most of the time.

I was diagnosed three years ago after 20 years of seeing many doctors and looking for answers. Due to my standard blood tests being normal, I was always told I was fine - until I persisted and got a diagnosis of ME/CFS/fibromyalgia. These were merely labels for my symptoms though. I felt they did not answer any question as to the cause of my symptoms.

I was lucky to find an excellent doctor (Professor Chris O'Callaghan; The University of Melbourne, Austin Hospital, Melbourne, Australia) who actually knew about EDS and POTS. He was able to describe and explain all my symptoms and diagnose me accurately. He did a tilt table test to diagnose POTS. I had no idea I had POTS/Orthostatic Intolerance as I had only fainted once as a teenager and did not get much dizziness. My palpitations had been helped with magnesium supplements and I did not connect many of my other symptoms with the condition. I believed that to have POTS you needed to feel constantly faint or dizzy. I learned, however, that some people can cope and their body adapts. This helps them stay upright for certain periods but then they experience symptoms and illness later. Professor O'Callaghan also took a full and thorough medical history – he asked about all my symptoms from childhood – and those of ALL my family members. This was repeated at the Connective Tissue Disorders section of the Genetics Department at the Royal Melbourne Hospital where my EDS diagnosis was later confirmed.

Once I had the diagnosis, I started to see the correlations, patterns and the strong family history; many in my family are also Gorlin's sign positive and a couple have Marfan's habitus.

What has been your greatest challenge in your health?

Fatigue, episodic brain fog (dyscognition) and IBS. Also PEM (post-exertional malaise) which means I get quite ill in subsequent days any time I exercise – even though I love to exercise.

What we call fatigue - I actually think it is orthostatic intolerance and crashing but fatigue is as close as we get in a word to describe it as two things happen: 1), you either feel the need to lie down because you are not getting enough blood to your brain when you are upright, or 2), you are suffering from the time you spent upright with brain fog and other severe debilitating symptoms and so you need to lie down to recover.

After I stand up for any length of time, I get severe payback symptoms in the following days which can, at its worst, be like having a bad hangover, a bad case of food poisoning, and the flu combined.

It is really a need to lie down because I don't get enough blood to my head when I stand up due to a combination of orthostatic intolerance, POTS, and low blood volume. I have low blood volume, which was tested for in a special blood test – a red cell mass test (also called a plasma volume test).

How have you changed because of your diagnosis?

I can see the logic in my symptoms and I can control or manage them better now.

I plan more if I want to do an outing and I recover better because I recognize what will help me recover and what will prevent recovery. I also monitor my oxygen saturations with a home pulse oximeter and found they are usually too low at home – about 89% to 91% most of the time when they should be 95% or above. I also use the oximeter to monitor my pulse and if it is too high due to POTS, I will take it a bit easier.

I know what to avoid - things like heat and alcohol - which are vasodilators and exacerbate my symptoms. I also avoid hot crowded rooms, supermarkets or any situations that involve prolonged standing. I now know all these things will make me ill and are likely exacerbate my insomnia that night. As a result, I modify these activities by ordering groceries online or shopping at off-peak times when there is no wait.

What is something you have overcome in your health?

I follow a low FODMAPS diet to help manage IBS symptoms and I take lactase capsules to control lactose intolerance. Managing these helps minimize the gut malabsorption, which, as Dr. Heidi Collins has pointed out, can result in us becoming malnourished, as we are not getting adequate vitamin and mineral absorption over many years. I also take a regular Vitamin C supplement – which seems to stave off the otherwise frequent infections I get due to EDS – and magnesium for the muscle tightness and cramps.

Did you have a major turning point? If so, what was it and how did your life change?

Getting the EDS/POTS diagnosis from Professor Chris O'Callaghan was the major turning point for me. Prior to that I felt I was at the mercy of my unpredictable symptoms. Dr. Jason Tye-Din (Royal Melbourne Hospital; Walter and Eliza Hall Institute) ruled out coeliac disease for me and diagnosed my fructose malabsorption and IBS which also helped me manage my symptoms better.

Finding the EDNF website was a big plus. They have lots of great information, which is updated regularly. I also found lots of YouTube clips and publications from many doctors including Dr. Clair Francomano, Dr. Heidi Collins, Dr. Brad Tinkle, Professor Rodney Grahame, Dr. Kaz Kaz, Dr. Marco Castori, Professor Chris O'Callaghan, Professor Peter Rowe, Dr. Alan Pocinki, and Dr. Anne Maitland. This changed my life by helping me to become informed and educated about my condition.

Connecting with fellow EDSers and POTSies through Facebook has been helpful, too. We all share our stories, problems, and solutions. I've met many fabulous and loyal friends there who encourage me when I'm down and share terrific medical information and articles that we can discuss. Even better is that there is always someone online around the clock, which is great if you suffer from insomnia. There's less social isolation this way.

How did overcoming that challenge change how you perceived your health?

I no longer try to push through. I realize this condition is permanent and that no amount of effort or determination is going to improve my health. Instead, I work within my limitations. For example, if I do not need to get up I will stay in bed and work on the laptop. This means I do not have my legs dangling down while I sit in a chair so I do not exacerbate my OI/POTS. This helps me to NOT feel extremely ill all the time.

What have you done to overcome low points throughout your journey?

When I am having a bad day, I recognize this, and try not to push myself. I stay in bed and use the laptop – connect with friends on Facebook, watch movies, or read if I am able. If necessary, I keep the room dark and quiet, hydrate well with electrolytes, and wear abdominal compression to relieve my symptoms. I use caffeine wisely in the mornings, as it is a vasoconstrictor, which can provide some relief, but keeps me awake, if I drink it in the afternoons. On a very bad day, I will drink an energy drink as the caffeine (which helps POTS because it is a vasoconstrictor) combined with a sugar hit can often alleviate some of the symptoms.

If you could offer one piece of advice to someone reading this book that felt disheartened by his or her diagnosis or health, what would you say?

There is always hope with magic of the Internet. We have increased speed of communication in medical research and advances in genetics – a combination that brings hope for a cure. The Internet is also a powerful tool to spread awareness and to educate others who have not yet connected the dots of their EDS, POTS, or MCAD symptoms. Many people are still misdiagnosed and seeking answers in Facebook groups. They have been told they have fibromyalgia, ME/CFS, anxiety disorders (POTS can mimic or cause these symptoms), Hashimoto's, autism and SPD (sensory processing disorders). When we educate others, we see more diagnoses. The more people who get diagnosed properly, the more attention we can generate to lobby for governments to change funding priorities.

The recent ALS ice bucket challenge raised over $100 million for research. This proves that the Internet is a powerful tool. But, we need to remember that AIDS did not receive attention or funding for research until people protested and demanded change. We must be proactive in our awareness campaigns.

Is there anything else that you would like to add that isn't covered in the answers above?

I am still keen to try intravenous therapy to treat my low blood volume and POTS. I would also like to try intranasal oxygen therapy to see if it helps my low oxygen saturations. I am researching both of these treatments and watching the Vanderbilt University Study for outcomes on low blood volume in POTS.

I think I am lucky to have an EDS diagnosis because I know my mother had identical symptoms and never even found out what was wrong with her. She spent the last 20 years of her life confined to bed without answers. All her life she knew there was something wrong but never found out what it was or met anyone with the same issues to discuss them with. While she never was diagnosed, I find hope that I have a diagnosis and can be proactive in my care.

One positive thing you can say about Ehlers-Danlos syndrome it that is an extremely interesting disease. Because connective tissue is all throughout the body EDS causes a vast array of symptoms. So studying it is never boring. I like facts, learning about my conditions, and putting the pieces of the puzzle together. One of the first things I did after diagnosis was to start a thread of information for others so they could not only learn about EDS (and the comorbidities), but also know what steps they can take to receive a proper diagnosis.

As I navigated many Facebook groups, I noticed that many doctors were saying to patients, "You might have EDS, but it does not really matter. It is not going to make a difference." It was because of this that I compiled 20 Reasons to Get an Ehlers-Danlos Syndrome Diagnosis.

WHY bother to get an EDS diagnosis?

How will that help me? – 20 Good Reasons
1. EDS is genetic so you may want to know for your kids/ grandkids who may get it worse than you - and to avoid passing it on if you plan on kids.
2. There are associated cardiovascular risks so you need to have an echocardiogram every 5 years - for all types of EDS especially to rule out aortic arch issues.
3. It is a great relief if you get a diagnosis because, when you understand it, it explains all your symptoms logically and you do not feel like you are crazy, depressed, and anxious or have social phobias - EDS has physical reasons for all of these.
4. Experts estimate that one in every 100 people have EDS but are just undiagnosed - if we all get diagnosed and the huge numbers with EDS are realized we will get more research and a possible cure.
5. There are great symptomatic management strategies for it once you know what you are dealing with - and getting a correct diagnosis is a basic right.
6. You can connect with others who have it too which is a great relief and a good source of information.
7. You should be aware of pregnancy risks such as postpartum hemorrhage and miscarriages.
8. There are dental issues like poor teeth, dental crowding and periodontitis that you may want to take extra care over - EDSers often need more local anesthetic for dental procedures, for example.
9. Sometimes it helps you realize what other symptoms you DO have - e.g. you may not know what brain fog is until you read about it as I did and it clicks - "oh yes, that is those days when I lie in bed all day and can do nothing and feel like I have a hangover for no reason"...same with heat intolerance - why you are worse in the heat; photophobia (sensitivity to light), hyperacusis (sensitivity to noise), etc.
10. There are many eye issues associated with EDS such as nearsightedness, detached retina and keratoconus so you may want to let your optometrist/ophthalmologist know about it and investigate these.
11. It can help if you are giving up smoking to know that nicotine is a stimulant and part of the reason you feel bad when you try to stop smoking is that smoking seems to mask some of your EDS symptoms so you feel better when you smoke....ditto for caffeine which is a vasoconstrictor.... so if you are addicted to cola drinks.....POTS or EDS may be part of the reason.
12. Some of the symptoms - brain fog, crashes, can feel like depression when they seem to hit "out of the blue" - these can be relieved by treatments

such as rehydrating with electrolytes, wearing compression garments, etc. maybe you do not have depression after all....

13. EDS can help explain seemingly unrelated issues involving multiple body systems. Also why an injury can seem to "move" from one joint to another (e.g. you splint your wrist, and it may cause problems in the neighboring joints - e.g. thumb and elbow because all the joints are susceptible to overuse injuries.)

14. You can get appropriate management with knowledgeable healthcare providers (e.g. physios who know about joint hypermobility and what kinds of treatments to do/exercises to give) and learn joint protection strategies. And you can avoid unnecessary treatments and tests.

15. EDS can predispose you to allergies that can lead to a risk or possibility of anaphylaxis.

16. EDS is now being linked to MCAD (mast cell activation disorder), which for many is treatable with new protocols that bring great symptomatic relief (e.g. Zyrtec/Zantac combo).

17. Another one of the symptoms is dysphagia (or difficulty swallowing) and choking on fluids, food or sometimes just your saliva - this of course can also be potentially very dangerous.

18. This point is from Dr. David Chorley: "Oh and I just thought of a real life example from my own medical practice (yes I'm a doctor who knows about EDS): A significant number of EDS patients have blood clotting problems, so I have initiated my own protocol of screening teenage EDS women for Protein C+S, Antithrombin III, Factor V Leiden and homocysteine. Out of my 150 EDS patients I have found about 10 with defects. This is huge because if a young woman goes on Birth Control Pill with a clotting disorder she can have a stroke or myocardial infarct."

19. Anyone with EDS should totally AVOID fluoroquinolone antibiotics, which can cause damage to connective tissues like tendons and ligaments.

20. AORTIC DISSECTION IS OFTEN MISSED AND MISDIAGNOSED AS A HEART ATTACK! (Sadly this happened with actor John Ritter.) EDS can also make you prone to aneurysms. This is why all types of EDSers need an echocardiogram at least every 5 years - to check the status of the aortic arch that can change over time.

WRITTEN BY CONTESSA COURTNEY

Contessa Courtney is a Division One Registered Nurse with over 20 years' experience in medical and surgical nursing, including intensive care, cardiac care, pediatrics, oncology, and palliative care..

For the last several years Contessa has been engaged in academic and medical research. She holds degrees from The University of Melbourne and La Trobe University, including a Master's Degree by research from The University of Melbourne. Her extensive research into ME/CFS/(SEID), fibromyalgia, EDS, POTS, MCAD and related conditions such as hypovolemia has been the focus of her research and attention for four years now.

She is actively engaged in promoting EDS, POTS and MCAD awareness and education and was recently invited to speak to medical students at The University of Melbourne on the first two of these research areas.

With the help and support of a wonderful and dedicated team of administrators and advisory members Contessa moderates several Facebook support groups whose combined memberships currently exceed 10,000. These groups provide education and first line support for people all around the world who have or are looking into EDS, POTS and MCAD diagnoses.

Her eclectic range of other interests include European languages and cinema, classical music, especially opera, cello and piano, gardening, painting in mixed media, and collecting textiles from all around the world.

Some of her Facebook groups are here:

EDS/ME/CFS/FM/POTS/OI articles and info
Stiff Zebras - EDS with joint or muscle stiffness
Ehlers-Danlos EDS/POTS Australia and International

Forum: **InvisibleIllnessForum.com**

Her blog: **RainbowZebraStampede.com**

REFLECTIONS

"Reflect upon your present blessings of which every man has many – not on your past misfortunes, of which all men have some." – Charles Dickens

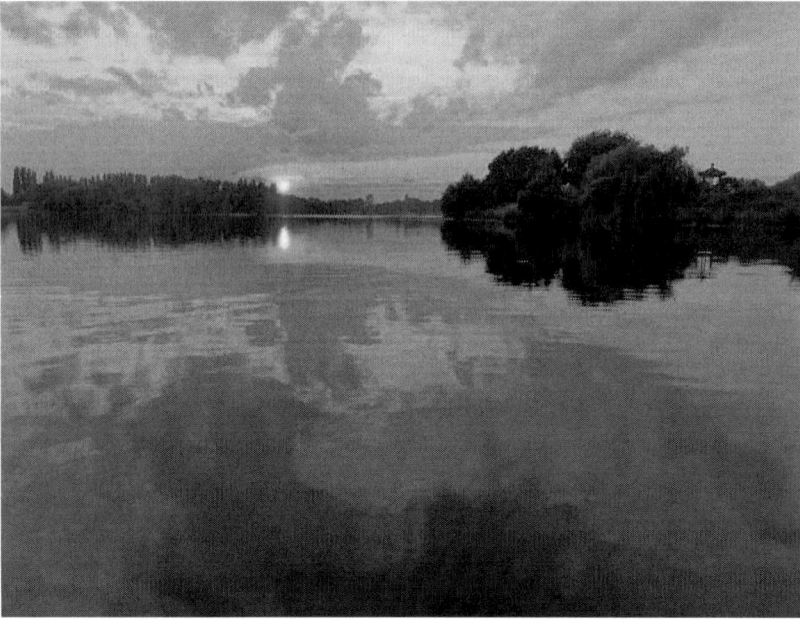

SOS

A Q&A with Kyle Leibe

What type of EDS do you have and when were you diagnosed?

My shoulder started dislocating first around 2001. I had reconstructive surgery in 2002 due to a torn bicep muscle and rotator cuff, and a severe slap lesion in the joint that occurred during my bi-annual physical fitness test in the military. During the test, as I rounded a corner running, my shoulder dislocated again. I kept running to finish the test, but then went to medical to be checked. My shoulder was totally blown and I was sent to Bethesda Naval Hospital and Walter Reed to see various specialists for reconstructive surgery. After my shoulder was repaired, I had numerous surgeries on my left knee because my kneecap kept popping out of place. I also damaged the cartilage on the femur. Through the various tests, and after the 3rd surgery on my left knee, the doctors decided to use cadaver parts to reconstruct my knee – everything else had failed. After that, I started questioning why so much was going wrong when I was still so young and in good shape.

I was having back issues due to a number of falls in the military. I found out that a disk was ruptured, another one was bulging and impinging the nerves, and part of my L5 vertebrae was broken. After that, I had to go in front of a medical review board in Washington, DC at the Navy Yard. The doctors who sat on the board did not understand why my body would be reacting to the various injuries and surgeries other than I must have broken my back prior to entering the military. (They had no idea about EDS and I was not diagnosed at the time.) . At that time, they deemed that the military was responsible for my knees, but that my back was broken prior to my service and they gave me an honorable medical discharge from the military. Unfortunately they provided only a severance package and no benefits or retirement for my 8 years of service.

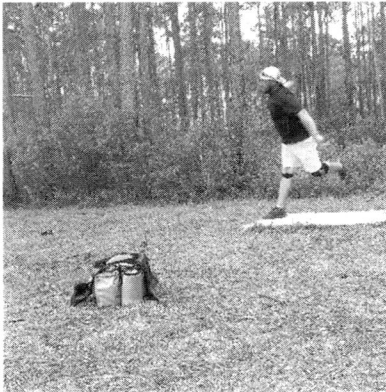

At the time I was also married with 2 kids and having a bunch of medical issues, mentally and physically exhausted, on a ton of pain meds, and had to start dealing with my back issues. However, the military acknowledged a problem with my back, but refused to treat it because they did not want to give me any more disability than I was already going to get. When I finally had my first spine fusion, my wife had already left me due to various life stressors and my medical issues. We remained amicable for the kids and I had already planned to stay with my best friend and his family after my surgery. During the stay in the hospital after my first spinal fusion, I asked my wife to bring my kids to see me. She ended up coming alone. In my hospital room, she was crying and telling me that she thought I was faking all of my problems, because I couldn't help much around the house and with the kids. I asked her to leave because there was no way I would be able to convince a doctor to do a spine fusion on me if I was faking it.

I left the hospital and recovered at my friend's house, during which, my mom came to help and discussed my issues with my friend's wife, Kendra. Kendra recommended that I go see the genetics department that she had been to for a proper evaluation for Ehlers-Danlos Syndrome. I was diagnosed with Classical EDS right after Kendra in 2006 through the genetics department at University of Maryland at the age of 27.

I had always shown signs of hypermobility. By the time I was diagnosed, I had been through 7 or 8 surgeries for various injuries. I always thought that my injuries and related surgeries were due to my service in the military because I was always in such good shape. When your body is so much stronger and fit, you don't notice all the signs of EDS. I didn't notice anything was wrong until after that first shoulder injury.

I now had a diagnosis that I hoped would help me find a way to get the best treatment for my various ailments. I still had to have two more spine fusion surgeries and five more surgeries on my knees in order to repair the damage that had been done up until that point. I decided to seek proper treatment outside of the military community, and paid for everything myself. The military physicians' lack of knowledge and willingness to learn about the complications and severity of issues associated with Ehlers-Danlos Syndrome was the driving force for this decision.

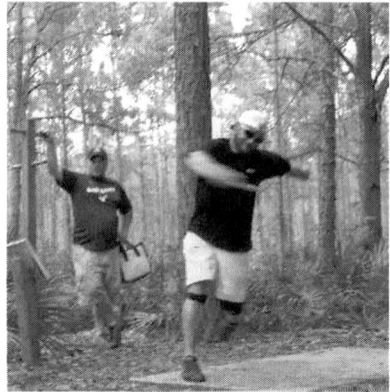

This was after 9/11 and the US was fully engaged in war in Afghanistan and Iraq. There were obviously many servicemen and servicewomen who were coming back from deployments with injuries, and cases like mine were pushed aside, despite the fact that I had also gotten hurt while serving my country.

The real issue is that because of security clearance, I cannot tell anyone how exactly I got hurt – what I did and the proper details to help someone understand my injuries.

At this point, I'm out of the military and working as a DoD contractor in the intelligence community in the DC area and have very good insurance. I was able to seek out care from the best doctors. I was able to have the two additional spine fusions needed and other knee surgeries by the Baltimore Ravens Ortho Group in Baltimore, MD. This surgeon researched EDS. He took the time to ask me questions about my specific case, and presented my case at a conference in San Diego with other orthopedic surgeons to help him approach my specific injuries with the best prognosis possible. He felt confident that his approach would have a positive outcome.

The last surgery was the most intense. I had my lower right leg cut in half just below the knee to realign the patella tendon and knee cap properly in my trochlear groove (knee joint). During this surgery, they also took part of my thigh, drilled holes around the kneecap, and wound the thigh through the kneecap securing it with a screw to prevent future dislocations. They also cut away the bad cartilage around and behind my knee cap, drilled numerous small holes and sewed a thin membrane over the entire area of lost cartilage. The surgeon injected that area with cord stem cells in order to grow new cartilage. It was the most brutal surgery I've ever had. I do not remember much from the two months following my surgery.

I stayed with friends following this surgery. I was in a wheelchair and the pain was awful. That was the last surgery I had because I was just done. I started looking into other treatment methods and ways to handle the pain. After another discussion with Kendra, I sought the care of one of the known EDS specialists in DC. He was understanding and approached my overall treatment from various angles versus just orthopedic. He recommended that I go on long-term disability from my employer because I was killing myself trying to work, go to school, see my kids, and have a life with the out-of-control spiral of my health. This physician also wanted to tackle associated EDS issues, such as sleep and autonomic dysfunction, in order to help manage compounding factors in my particular case and chronic pain. I felt hopeful after seeing him. I believed I could get things moving in the right direction and learned that there are doctors who do believe.

I went on disability and moved down to Florida. I lived with my parents so I could focus on regaining my strength and my life; for myself and my kids.

Since then, I've been dropped from Aetna for my long-term disability because they do not understand EDS and that it's not just pain or orthopedic issues; it's a true multi-systemic condition. In addition, I've been denied social security disability and I've been waiting on my claim with the VA for 6 years. The claim with the VA is for me to receive benefits for the injuries and disorders that I endured while serving in the military. When you enlist in the military with a prior condition and they still accepted you, but that condition was aggravated during your service, you are still eligible to receive benefits. Even though I was obviously born with EDS, I did not know about it until I was medically discharged. The military expected me to uphold my contract to serve my country; yet, they are not upholding their end of the contract by providing me the benefits that I deserve.

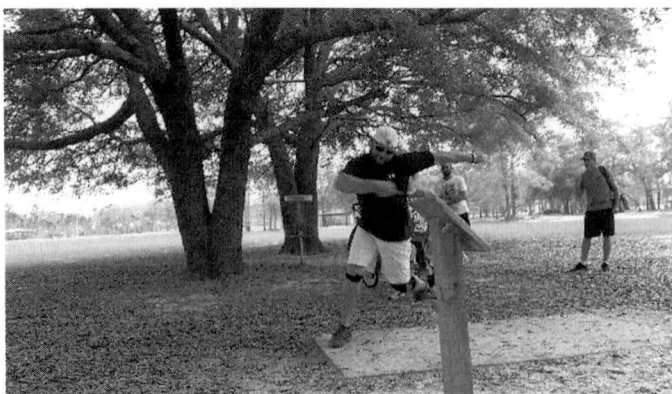

Right now, I'm still in Florida with my parents, I've started seeing mental health professionals due to post traumatic stress disorder (PTSD) as a result of the physical stress of having complications due to EDS, the mental and emotional stress that I've endured due to the trauma while serving, and because the government has failed to support one of their injured servicemen.

I've started a few new hobbies that help me stay active, while also being gentle on my body. In playing disc golf, I have been able to share my story with others. Through the enjoyment I have with this hobby and my desire to help others, I have started teaching a clinic on disc golf for wounded veterans under the Wounded Warrior Project. It allows me to share my love for disc golf and how this sport has saved my life, while remaining active both physically and within the military service community.

What has been your greatest challenge in your health?

Keeping my spirits up and remaining active with chronic pain and fatigue. Once I started dealing with PTSD, and the anxiety and depression that stems from it, I have been able focus on ways to help gain the strength that I need to keep my joints in place and manage life with chronic pain.

How have you changed because of your diagnosis?

Completely changed - life is short and doesn't always work out the way you want. Don't wait to do things that you want to do, just do them. If you are going to go down, go down swinging. If you can help someone else while you are you dealing with your own struggles, you gain strength, self-worth, and it makes you feel good.

Did you have a major turning point? If so, what was it and how did your life change?

Moving to Florida, moving in with my parents, and on disability with no income and nothing left to my name was a major turning point. I was divorced, had recently broken-up with my girlfriend of two years, had to stop going to school, couldn't work, had no car, was broke, and had no means to see my children.

In this, I realized that life wasn't about me and what I had, it's what can I do to help others who are dealing with similar situations like me. I still very much believe in the oath that I took to serve my country and to help others that can't help themselves, but I'm doing it in a different way now.

I don't pity the situation that I am in anymore. It is what it is. I just have to deal with it and change the way I treat my body. Keeping a positive mental mindset is absolutely crucial.

What have you done to overcome low points throughout your journey?

When you have a positive mindset, it allows you to change the things that you need to change and accept and deal with the things that you can't change. I can't change the fact that I have EDS, but I can change the way that I view life and not allow this condition to get me down anymore. I still have bad days or bad stretches, but as long as I'm able to live more on the positive side, then I am moving in the right direction.

If you could offer one piece of advice to someone reading this book that felt disheartened by his or her diagnosis or health, what would you say?

Get over it. Once you get over the fact that you can't change it, you can start working towards getting to your new normal… whatever your new normal is for you. When you have EDS, you will be forced to find a new normal; even in just your mindset if you are not that affected physically. The person I was in 2006 when I was diagnosed and even who I was in 2013 when I went on long-term disability, is a completely different person than I am now. When I was able to accept having EDS and that I can't change it, I was forced to change my mindset to strengthen my mind, body, and soul.

Is there anything else that you would like to add that isn't covered in the answers above?

Having someone who is close to you, who believes you and is willing to help, goes a long way. (Thanks Mom and Dad!)

What resolve have you gained for your own journey?

I'm going to continue to do what I like and enjoy life. Life is short and fragile. Losing a portion of me has helped me realize that there are still things I'm meant to do, want to do, and will still do. Nothing will stop me.

My goals are to be happy and help people. If I do that, everything else will fall into place.

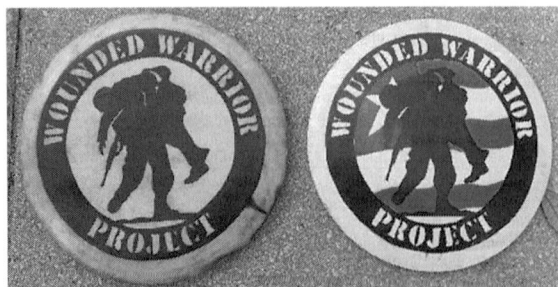

WRITTEN BY KYLE LEIBE

"It is an honor and a privilege to be of service and support; however, I realize people are not putting their confidence in me. Instead, they are actually learning to trust themselves. My job is to affirm and support them in the process and teach them to do what I do when I need strength: I begin within."
– Iyanla Vanzant

A Letter to Emily's Mom

Dear Emily's Mom,

Everything is going to be okay. Really, it is.

Yes, I know Emily - your baby girl - has Ehlers-Danlos Syndrome and it seems like the end of the world. I know she is only 11 years old and she is losing everything that matters and your heart is breaking for her and for yourself because your world has been unceremoniously turned upside down. Life as you knew it is a memory and a new life, an uncertain and daunting one, is looming.

Yes, I know she got EDS from her daddy and her brother has it too and you are thinking if only you had known when she was younger, maybe things wouldn't have to be this bad for her. You are also feeling relief to finally have answers about all the strange symptoms she has had since she was a baby, while simultaneously knowing that relief is a bizarre emotion to be feeling with such a diagnosis.

Yes, I know you are terrified. I know you feel utterly unqualified to deal with this, guilty for not knowing sooner, and heartbroken to see your daughter suffering so. I know you can't see where this path will lead and I know you hate not being in control.

Five years down the trail from where you sit now, broken and grieving at the beginning of the journey, I can see where you are going and where I have been. Which is why I can say, with certainty that everything is going to turn out fine. Truly it is.

Take a moment to breathe and absorb that truth. *Everything is going to be okay.*

That belief will be sorely tested in the days to come. You are going to have moments where you doubt, where you will not be able to see down the path you are on; moments where it won't seem possible that the world will ever be right again. But, everything is going to be okay.

I promise.

Of course, "everything is going to be okay" doesn't mean things will be easy or that events will fall out according to your liking. Spoiler Alert: events will very rarely, if ever, fall out according to your liking. Honestly, what you think should happen is not always what needs to happen and that will be a hard lesson to learn... One of many hard lessons you will learn, I hate to say.

Somehow, though, even when things don't go your way, things still turn out okay. When I say, "everything will be okay," what I mean is that, even in the most difficult circumstances, you will be able to honestly say, "it is well with my soul." You won't get there overnight, but you **will** get there.

Faith is at the heart of this journey and it will be your greatest weapon against all of the challenges and uncertainty you face. You will learn that you aren't in control, no matter how much you want to be, and that you can either be driven crazy by that or simply believe that God has more knowledge than you do so you can trust his plans for you. The circumstances you face are going to make you more vulnerable and more adrift than you have ever been and you will survive by leaning heavily on the promise in Romans that tells of how God is working to make all things – even EDS – good. What's more, you will see that promise come true, time and time again. Soon, you will even come to see the journey as a gift.

Believe it or not, you are being given the amazing opportunity to become more…

More faithful. More patient. More compassionate. More real. More human. You will have the privilege of making friends and meeting people who you otherwise never would have met – in a hidden world of people suffering from invisible, chronic illness will be revealed to you and you will be blessed by that revelation and by them.

You will learn the beauty of service: both serving the ones you love and being served by others who care about you. You will gain knowledge and have experiences that will shape you as a human being; a better human being than you were before. You will weep and laugh, pray and think, and learn and grow. It will be painful and profound, but you will find your purpose on this planet and you will grow in love and compassion. This whole crazy <u>awful</u> business is a precious opportunity to evaluate your priorities, shore up relationships and get rid of all the unnecessary stuff in your life.

No, I know it doesn't feel like an opportunity right now, it feels more like a punishment. But you aren't being punished! Rain falls on the righteous and the unrighteous alike. You will witness God working through those bad things and transforming them into something beautiful. And, trust me, the beauty will come. Just watch for it. It will come in big, spectacular ways; in tiny, gentle whispers; and though rainbows peeking through the storm clouds. It will come…

Now, I won't lie… this journey you are on will not be easy. When I talk of the beauty to come, it might be hard to believe when the darkness is pressing in on all sides. Those moments are real and it is okay to despair, to grieve, to doubt – give yourself permission to feel whatever it is that you feel. You don't have to always see the beauty of the journey – there are parts of it that are just plain hard. When things are rough, just cling to the hope that beauty will be coming during those dark times. That hope will be your anchor.

You are facing the fight of your life - there is no point in sugar coating it. From my vantage point, way down the road from where you are, I can look back and see the steep, rocky trail ahead of you, the pitfalls, the detours, the sleepless nights and the awful times when you are just going to have to sit tight and be patient. However, I can also see the molding of your character and the resilience that comes from the hard work of walking the path you are on. I can also see the beauty being wrought from the ashes and the rainbows that have been scattered along the way.

From your vantage point, at the starting line of this marathon, you see only the unknown and it is terrifying. You have every right to be afraid. In fact, fear will be a tool to harness on your journey, but what you need to know is that fear, in the end, is not what will define your journey. **Love is**.

I know you will struggle to believe this in the beginning, but the destination is worth the challenges of the journey. The journey will not destroy you. It will make you stronger than you ever thought you could be. You and yours will not only survive this journey – you will thrive.

Here's another Spoiler Alert: Emily is alright. More than alright, in fact.

She is an amazing young lady. She is not defined nor defeated by her diagnosis. She has faced some pretty tough times and is a fierce fighter – you call her your hero and she has earned that title. And, tough as she is, she still has love and compassion aplenty. She is strong, smart, talented and funny. Your fears that she would not be able to withstand this challenge are completely unfounded. Just as your character is being shaped by this journey, so, too, is hers. And, while you wish she could be free from troubles, you know that is just the wishful thinking of a parent. EDS is simply part of her life and she is learning to rise admirably to the challenges that she will face for the rest of her life.

Sure, there is the day-to-day EDS stuff to deal with – the dislocations, injuries, the pain, the headaches, the autonomic stuff. Unfortunately, those never go away. But, somehow, you both will adapt to all of that and learn to roll with it. Like I said, EDS does not define nor defeat her or you, for that matter.

You will find some good medical care along the way and you will find that a willingness to think outside the box will serve you well. Family, friends, and faith will keep you strong. You will make mistakes but when you do you will learn from them and you will hone your knowledge to become a formidable advocate. And your daughter will learn how to advocate for herself from your example.

Long story short: you can do this.

I am still looking towards an unknown future so I can't tell you how the journey ends. We have a long way to go and I have no crystal ball from here on out. What I can tell you, with confidence, is that, while I fully expect troubles because troubles are part of life, I also have confidence that there will be rainbows that accompany the storms, weeping will turn to joy, God's mercies are new each morning and beauty will come from the ashes of the most difficult situation. So, whatever troubles are lurking around the next bend in the road, I know we will be alright.

And so will you.

Hang in there,

Beth (Emily's Mom)

WRITTEN BY BETH SMITH

Beth blogs about her family's journey with EDS at Our Lives with Ehlers-Danlos Syndrome. She is mom to Lucas and Emily, wife to Andrew and is blessed by her family of Zebras. When she is not writing, she enjoys reading and theatre.

Beth blogs about their journey in living with EDS from a parent's perspective at: **SlingsAndArrowsOfOutrageousFortune.wordpress.com**

Climbing Joshua Tree

Sometimes I truly impress myself, especially in those moments when I gracefully accomplish something identified as "impossible." One of the most significant lessons I have learned from living with Ehlers-Danlos Syndrome is that it's not that I am unable to do certain things; rather, it's a matter of getting the proper training, equipment, and support system to conquer anything I set my mind to. It's interesting to think about the word impossible - it literally spells out "I'm possible!" This just goes to show how overcoming even the greatest challenges all comes down to a matter of perspective.

Weeks after being diagnosed with Ehlers-Danlos Syndrome, I met a fellow EDSer who had just completed a marathon; a feat others said was "impossible" with her condition. Our brief conversation left a profound impact on me; she said something I will never forget: "If we all did the things we were truly capable of, it would literally astound us."

This interaction made me re-evaluate the things I previously thought to be possible and impossible for myself as an individual living with EDS. I decided to no longer allow the limiting beliefs of physicians hold me back from living a life full of passion and success. I made a conscious decision to see that each day would bring about new adventures. I committed to finding creative ways to get myself over the hurdles of my condition, and embrace these adventures to the fullest.

One of the greatest, most challenging adventures I've had to embrace was learning to walk again after a failed L5-S1 fusion surgery.

Seven years ago, every intake of oxygen left my lungs aching, and every step was profoundly painful. The reality of that situation was I would often be confined by immobility, stuck in my bed for hours, days, weeks, and sometimes months. I became so physically and emotionally debilitated that on a bad day, just gathering the strength to get out of bed to go to the bathroom was an impressive feat within itself. When the pain became too much to handle, I left college and moved home in search of answers.

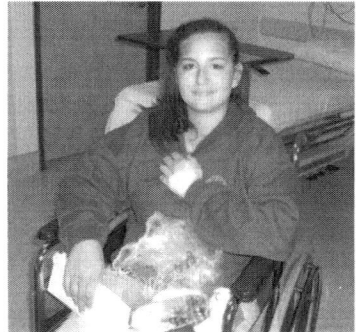

My wonderfully supportive parents believed in me, my strength, and my potential - even when I didn't believe in myself. They found an extraordinary practitioner, Brian Danek, who created a strict nine hour a day, seven days a week, wellness plan. He showed me a variety of constructive techniques to alleviate the pains I was experiencing, offering a solution beyond a medical prescription. With the help of my support system, in spite of the seemingly endless challenges EDS brings, my body's physical functionality improved slowly.

Overtime, I was able to take my first steps without pain. This was something previously believed to be "impossible" in my world. I had resigned to living a life filled with pain, unaware that if I changed my lifestyle, my symptoms would change as well. Each day, I continue to achieve more of these small steps toward wellness. However, getting to this point did not come easily.

Overcoming a daily battle with my home's staircase was my first goal when I moved home. My bedroom was on the second floor of our home, which made it especially difficult to access given my situation. At that point, taking steps without causing additional agonizing pain was a major accomplishment. Walking up a staircase just to go to bed seemed like an impossible mission at first, as if I were climbing Mount Everest. However, over time it became easier as all things do with the proper training, focus, and dedication.

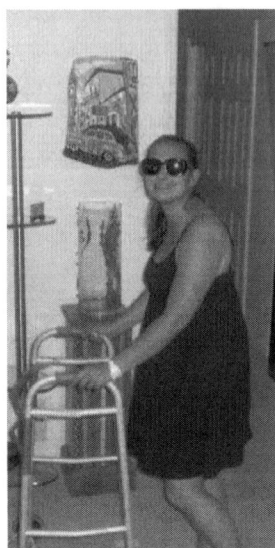

With each passing week, as I followed Brian's wellness plan, my body became stronger and stronger. He enforced steady increases in my physical activity and encouraged me to track my progress. Unfortunately, regardless of method, the healing process does not happen overnight. Although I was seeing positive results from this rigorous wellness program, by the end of each day, I was both physically and emotionally drained. I often used my very last bits of energy to climb the stairs to get into bed. The rest of the evening would be a blur of agonizing pain and chronic fatigue.

Brian's only request for the time between when he left at 5 pm and arrived the next morning at 8 am was that I walk for ten minutes. Sometimes, I would be confined to my room, too weak to move my body, yet desperately needing to. My parents, again, found a creative solution by putting a treadmill in my bedroom.

I truly believe this jump-started my love affair with walking. I remember taking pictures of the screen each day and texting them to my parents – "I walked for three minutes!"

"I walked for another four minutes!!!" a few hours after that.

Two hours later: "I walked another three minutes and completed my commitment for today! Ten minutes! Maybe I'll shoot for eleven minutes tomorrow!!" and so on until over time I could walk for longer. I had the mindset that it didn't matter if I wasn't strong enough to walk for ten minutes at one time, I still needed to do it even if it took me several hours.

I strove to master getting around our home, up and down the stairs – sometimes multiple times in a single day. During this time, I was able to understand that making conscious decisions to care for my body, such as eating healthfully or exercising, would affect my fortitude throughout my lifetime. I began to notice a new strength within my mind and body.

With each passing week, I became physically and emotionally stronger, in spite of the many challenges of living with EDS that appeared just as frequently. I even began to venture outside, something that took a lot of energy just a short time before. I still used a handicapped placard or tried to park in the closest spot to ensure that I could take as few steps as possible, but did so with the intention of accomplishing whatever errand was necessary; walking to and from the car was difficult on its own, never mind walking around and carrying things. But with time, patience, and practice, I was able to conquer these challenges as well.

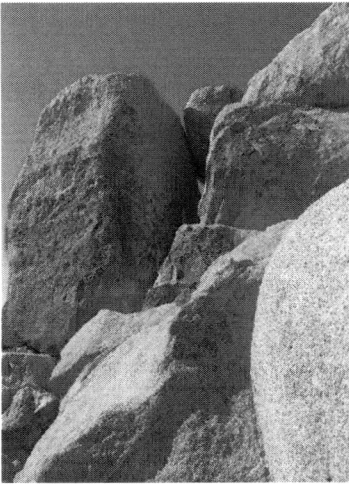

These victories may seem small, but each one merits just as much celebration as the last. In order to keep myself from becoming discouraged, it became essential to keep in mind that strength is not achieved overnight. I had to be committed to the process to see the benefits.

Even now that I have overcome many of those obstacles and live a life defined by wellness, I continue to track my strengths and weakness. I take pictures of the progress and the challenges so I am able to grow and learn from each. They serve as bookmarks of my progress. I once shied away from the camera, rarely allowing any documented evidence of my challenges before the age of 11. The few snapshots I do have from over the years have become an important part of my EDS journey. In the moments when I've come so far that I forget how sick I used to be, one glance at a photo from the past and I'm immediately propelled into action to continue my wellness journey.

To this day, I maintain my love affair with walking. In 2014, I walked 818 miles! After I conquered walking, I wanted to conquer hiking. I love the outdoors and learning to hike seemed like the perfect next step on my journey to wellness. After I conquered hiking, I wanted to conquer climbing. The desert provided an environment where I found inspiration surrounded by the natural world. After spending much time on hikes, I was ready to approach my newest challenge: climbing giant boulders at Joshua Tree National Park.

It was amazing. On the day I finally decided to climb, the sun was particularly harsh, beating down on my forehead with intimidating heat. Giant boulders stood tall around me, forming etched structures that lined themselves clumsily along the edges of Joshua Tree. A rigid rock jutted out from the boulder in front of where I stood. It formed a hold that was shaped perfectly to cradle my climbing shoes.

I stepped up and felt along the rough surface, sliding my fingers across the face of the boulder until my hand found a home in a crevice. I tucked my fingers into the rock's face and, making sure to balance my weight eased my body off the dirt floor and climbed up the first boulder.

As the distance between my body and the ground grew, I felt the fear building up inside causing a sudden limit to my breathing. I was hanging from the boulder's edge filled with terror, realizing I had only myself to rely on. Here, I was completely dependent on the strength of my own body to hold me up - the same body that couldn't even make it up a single stair not so many years ago.

In order to avoid a dangerous fall, I had to trust my strength, my muscles, my limbs, and most importantly, my breath. I could not allow self-doubt to take over. I had come too far. After confronting the presence of my fear, I shifted my mindset and smiled. I embraced the fear by accepting its authenticity and reminded myself that fear and excitement are chemically the same thing in your brain. By making the decision to remain excited and grateful for my body's ability to continue progressing on this journey, I was able to push myself up to exactly where it needed to be. I trusted my intuition, stayed focused, kept breathing, and eventually reached the top of the first massive boulder!

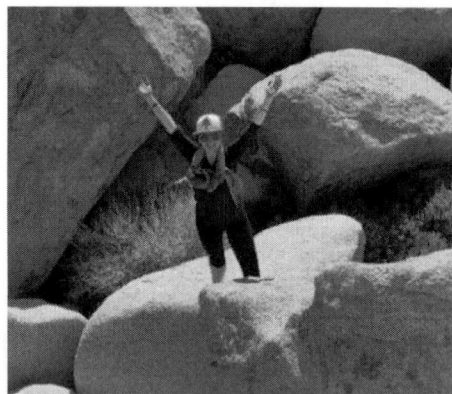

As I stood there, filled with amazement and pride, I soaked in the grandeur of my natural surroundings. I went on to climb the next one, and each time I reached the top of a new rock, I saw another that could be climbed. In succession, I climbed higher and higher on these massive boulders, culminating at the top where I realized that nothing was impossible any more – even when living with Ehlers-Danlos Syndrome.

WRITTEN BY BRIANNA GREENSPAN

Brianna Greenspan, a 27-year-old Ehlers-Danlos Syndrome (EDS) patient from California by way of Texas, is on a journey from illness to wellness. While she once lived a life defined by pain, she now lives a life driven by passion. One of Brianna's greatest passion is to help others find their own sense of strength and purpose. She believes everyone has a higher calling in life, but in order to achieve the best sense of self, one needs the necessary resources and the right the support system and resources.

Brianna strives to be a resource for the invisible illness community and currently, works as a wellness coach and consultant. Through her social media presence, and various other projects, Brianna hopes to propagate the idea that the labels other people impose do not define a person; everyone can be strong if they choose to be. Brianna Greenspan continues to pose as a leader for establishing wellness within the EDS community. Her upcoming book Back 2 Health: A patient and practitioners guide on the journey from illness to wellness, will offer an in-depth view of various approaches and a spectrum of modalities to help EDS patients gather information, communicate their needs, and get the help they require to live a life of wellness rather than disability.

Follow her on Instagram @drbri1111 or find her **Facebook**. (Brianna's Medical Journal) To learn about future updates and to find out about her upcoming book, visit: Back2HealthCommunity.com

Your time is limited, so don't waste it living someone else's life. Don't be trapped by dogma – which is living with the results of other people's thinking. Don't let the noise of others' opinions drown out your own inner voice. And most important, have the courage to follow your heart and intuition. – Steve Jobs

I Think I Might Be A Martian

"My arms feel like they might fall off," I said. "You're a nut!" my husband scoffed. I persisted, but he just rolled his eyes.

Over the years, we had scores of similar conversations, never realizing what they foreshadowed - that I unknowingly suffered from an invisible illness that was to profoundly affect our lives. Despite a vaguely uneasy sense of my limbs not being securely fastened to my body, and a collection of odd but minor quirks, I enjoyed excellent health, regularly hiking for miles and practicing yoga.

Then when I was about forty-seven years old, everything changed. After a few minor strains, my back mysteriously became so fragile that virtually any movement resulted in injury, and nothing helped. I could not drive, wash dishes or sit for an hour without long-term consequences. I ended up confined to bed while my husband wore himself out working and caring for me.

We consulted one doctor after another who merely gaped incredulously at my symptoms. Those who didn't throw up their hands often persuaded us to expend our limited time and financial resources on ineffective and sometimes harmful treatments.

After a while, my husband started calling me a Martian since the doctors here on Earth were clearly unfamiliar with my physiology. Lacking a better explanation, I wondered for the first time in my life whether I would be all right.

Then one day in a humble office on the outskirts of Silicon Valley, a rheumatologist barraged me for over an hour with seemingly unrelated questions about everything from my vision to my skin. With growing excitement, she had me touch my thumbs to my wrists, bend my fingers, elbows and knees backward, and place my hands flat on the floor (all of which I could do.)

At last, bursting with pride, she announced that I suffered from a genetic disorder I had never heard of called Ehlers-Danlos Syndrome. I was more fragile than others and at risk for a myriad of health problems. There was no treatment and no cure. Though this was hardly encouraging news, it served as a valuable epiphany, instantly connecting the dots between all my mysterious quirks as well as the storied medical history of my grandmother, previously dismissed as an epic hypochondriac.

Moreover, as we left the doctor's office, my husband of seventeen years finally conceded, "You weren't kidding when you said your arms felt like they might fall off." A wave of healing validation instantly surged through my genetically impaired body. Though we now know the scientific term for my condition, my husband continues to call me a Martian.

While the diagnosis supplied confidence, it fell far short of a solution. Largely unfamiliar with EDS, most health care professionals continued to be of little use. However, gradually through trial and error and the help of an exceptional physical therapist named Katrina, four helpful elements emerged: swimming and gentle warm water exercise, restorative sleep, medication to control pain, and adaptive strategies to avoid injury.

Within a year or two I made a remarkable recovery and felt I had been given a second chance. Just being able to drive to the grocery store was thrilling. To celebrate I went to the SPCA on my forty-eighth birthday and adopted an elegant looking, six-month-old, mixed breed puppy. I named her Chloe, and she became my loyal hiking companion. The next three years were the happiest of my life. Chloe and I spent countless hours joyfully exploring the spectacular local forests and hills of Central California. Thriving on abundant exercise, I grew healthy and fit while she bloomed into her prime.

Sadly this bright period was not to last. One day I made the mistake of doing just a few too many forward bends at a yoga class and re-injured my back. In a downward spiral I progressively lost everything I had gained and more, finally ending up confined to bed unable to drive, walk around the block, or lift a pillow without hurting myself. I could not even sit long enough to go out to dinner on special occasions. My husband grew overwhelmed, and friends were abruptly occupied with other priorities. We felt abandoned by the human race. Chloe, who could not understand why our happy jaunts in the woods had come to a crashing halt, languished on her bed engulfed in a funk. I could not even look at her without crying.

Then the phone rang. It was a fellow hiker, a woman with the unlikely name of Lloyd, whom I had encountered on the trails but hardly knew. All by herself, seeking neither compensation nor recognition, this extraordinary woman had been regularly walking dogs belonging to other ailing people. She called her canine hiking group the Muttley Crew, and with my undying gratitude, Chloe was invited to become its newest member. Seeing the smile return to Chloe's face boosted my spirits and allowed me to confront the most difficult time of my life with renewed motivation.

Soon afterward my husband arrived home from work beaming with excitement. A long-time customer had inquired how he was, and instead of the usual polite "Fine, thank you," he had shared the reality of our situation. Her reaction was as generous as it was immediate. Her name was Genie and she offered me, a total stranger, a weekly ride to the therapy pool. I was stunned. Later, I was equally surprised to discover that yet another angel had been quietly living next door for years. On learning of our difficulties, my neighbor Barbara also unexpectedly offered a weekly ride to the therapy pool.

These remarkable women, who have become dear friends, took me to the pool religiously while my husband continued shouldering the burden of my care. But this time I was not improving. Between feeble attempts to stay active, I lay in bed in discomfort. My back felt like a raw sore, and my once fit body withered and ached from tension and inadequate exercise. I did not get a good night's sleep for three years. Unable to go out, I stopped reading the calendar of events in the newspaper. Chloe's muzzle faded to gray while I doubted we would ever again walk through the woods together. Grief over the active, joyful life I had lost gradually displaced hope.

Despite waning expectations, I continued making adjustments to the multitude of strategies I had been trying and then amazingly began to get results. I modified my exercises, soaked in a hot bath before bed, figured out other ways to sleep better, tried a topical anti-inflammatory, and started getting massages from students at the local college. Step by step, I regained the ability to drive, cook simple meals, and enjoy fun outings. After three years without a good day, I could hardly believe I actually felt like myself again.

The other day, I achieved a milestone, taking Chloe for a two-mile walk in the woods where we encountered Lloyd. Beaming with delight, she told me later that we both had the most joyful smiles on our faces. On Thursday my husband and I celebrated the first Thanksgiving in a long time where we felt we truly had much for which to be thankful. Most of all, I am grateful to my husband Peter and my three angels Lloyd, Genie, and Barbara who have helped a Martian feel welcome on this earth.

WRITTEN BY THE MUSE OF COMEDY

Following a seventeen-year career as a certified public accountant, the Muse of Comedy is currently cultivating her true nature as a creative. She enjoys photography, graphic arts, and origami. She lives in California with her husband and dog. She has joint hypermobility EDS. Follow The Muse of Comedy on her blog: **StretchyGenes.wordpress.com**

Dedicated to my husband, Peter, and my three angels, Barbara, Lloyd, and Genie.

What EDS Means to Me

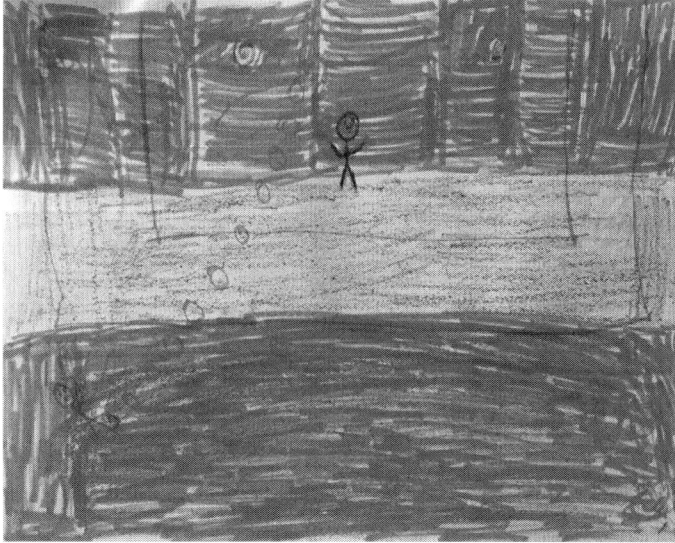

What does your picture represent?

Meaning is: Don't be afraid of having EDS and having to stop doing things that you want to do.

I saw kids at the EDNF conference that seemed to be giving up, because they wouldn't participate in the fun activities that we did and they would just sit out and not want to do anything. They didn't seem to want to do anything   because maybe they were afraid or didn't think that they could have fun because they had EDS. Some kids talked about knowing that they would end up in a wheelchair when they were older and that made me sad, because I didn't understand why they would say that.

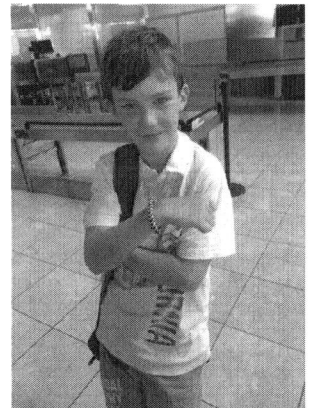

What do you think EDS is?

A syndrome that some people get and doctors are still trying to figure it out and there are 3 stages of it. Some can be very serious and some barely affect you. For example, there could be someone in a wheelchair and then there could be someone that seems barely affected.

I learned that there are ways to help yourself by staying active, drinking a lot water and choosing the right foods like Kefir (or "pro-bug") to help with congestion in your stomach.

What did you learn about giving back by going to EDNF conference & helping with charity ride by making bracelets?

It feels really good inside, because it makes people happy, raises awareness and I like hearing how much people like my bracelets. It cheers me up to want to make more.

What would you say to a kid who you met who had EDS or was just diagnosed and possibly was sad about having it?

I would make sure that I was friendly and share what my mom does, play with them at recess, and say "Hi!" when I see him/her.

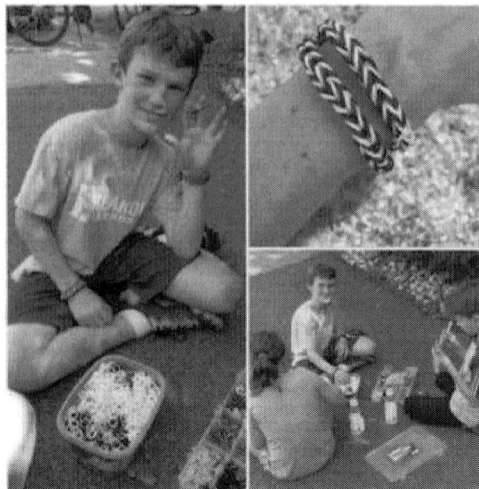

AS TOLD BY JOHANN MYLES

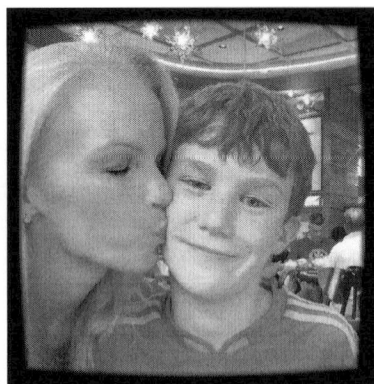

Johann is an active 10 year old who plays lacrosse, soccer, basketball, and his greatest love is ice hockey. He also sings in the church choir. Johann has not been formally diagnosed. His parents have made the decision to abstain from formal diagnosis after consulting with EDS specialists. His parents have handled the symptoms as they come with great success.

Normality

Normality is a crime. Normality is something that engulfs us, invades a person's mind taking over raiding everything in sight. Nothing can consume a person like normality. What does is it mean to be normal? The Merriam-Webster dictionary, defines normal as simply usual or ordinary: not strange. Although definable, what does the world normal really mean and why does it even matter?

Normal is not as simple as the dictionary says. Normal is not simply five words; it is so much more. It is an expectation set up by a society – a standard that we are all forced to achieve. Normality is the grey in a world full of color. Although this is true, to the majority of people, normality is a comfort. Society exerts an unnecessary amount of pressure for this one word. Everyone is put into a crucible, under pressure and heat until we all melt together… No longer recognizable and no longer ourselves. My only question about this is "Why?" Why can't we just go our own ways, be our own persons? Why do people judge, stare, and hate? Why is normality so important to so many people and what does it even mean? Although that is a question that, for me, will always be a mystery; I cannot help myself trying to imagine what it is like to be normal.

Once upon a time, I think I was normal. I had bleach blonde hair and lived mainly with my Grandmother. No one inspired me more than her. We used to sing and dance together, our favorite song being Favorite Things from The Sound of Music. I was five and my dream was that someday, I would go on to become a movie star. A friend and I even started saving in a piggy bank to move to Hollywood.

I was so happy. I always had a smile on my face. Life consisted of going around with my grandmother, doing all kinds of fancy things, and playing with my friends every chance I had. Life was simple and beautiful. I was normal… Then I got sick and my world was turned upside down.

I was six years old sitting alone at the playground because I had "weird" bumps on my skin. "She's weird!" "She's different!" They would point and stare. If one day I was sicker than the day before, I was suddenly faking. The words "Faker" and "Weirdo" all became common adjectives used to describe me. I went from singing and dancing to crying myself to sleep. I was alone. It felt as though there was no one there.

All these scary things were happening to me and none of my doctors knew why or what to do about them. The doctors told my mom that I was dislocating my shoulder for attention, and if she paid any attention to me she would make the problem worse by giving me what I wanted. The doctors told my Mom it just didn't make sense why a perfectly healthy girls shoulders would dislocate so easily on their own, so it must have been me pulling them out of place. My mom believed what the doctors were saying and it seemed as though everyone else did too. My mom constantly told me I was lying and asked me to stop getting sick, as if it was my choice. "Stop dislocating your shoulder." She would say. "Why do you have to do this, it's not fair to the rest of us." Her words piercing into me like knives that hurt more than the already existent pain. To me, it seemed like I spent my childhood fighting to survive, fighting to be heard and acknowledged. Constantly fighting for so many things, just yelling at the ceiling and waiting to be heard. No matter what the doctors or my mom said, I would never give up on that one word, that one thing which I wanted more than anything else, a normal life. I looked at all the other kids. I looked at them with a fiery envy that pulsated through my veins like a poison. More than anything, I wanted to be like them, and more than anything I wanted people to try to understand.

More than anything;

I wanted to run.
I wanted to play.
I wanted to walk.
I wanted to do things on my own.

I wanted to be free from this wheelchair, which tied me down constantly keeping me from living my life. I wanted to be just like them. I walked around with slings on my arms, being stared at everywhere I went, to anyone it was obvious I was never going be like the other kids. I still kept hoping. Although, it never mattered what I wanted because no matter how much I wanted to be normal, deep down I knew I could never be.

Through eight years, four extra diagnoses, eleven surgeries, and countless missed moments I have had to watch life go on while I was stuck at home. Although I look normal, I live every day in pain. Normal for me is anything but typical. My definition of normal is going to the ER at least once a month, a migraine every day, subluxations and dislocations, missing out on everything, pain and pills, more pain and more pills, and finally, having surgery about as often as I buy a new pair of shoes. I live anything but an ordinary life. To normal people, my life seems wild and scary, but I could never imagine living their normal.

People will tell me "Well you couldn't function with a migraine. So you must not have as bad of a headache as you say you do." The thing is, every day I am miserable. Every day I choose whether or not I should eat because I am constantly nauseated. I can barely listen in class because my head constantly feels like it is going to implode. People fail to see my pain because I choose to live my life in spite of pain.

I choose to get myself out of bed in the morning. I choose to go out with friends even though I slur my words because it hurts to talk.

For a while, I spent all my time in bed.
For a while, I spent my time with a washcloth over my head.
For a while I gave into my pain, I let my pain win.

My life became non-existent and I was a recluse. The thing is, after a while, I realized I can either live my life or I can watch it go by.

This is my life. This is my choice.

Normality is a crime. Normality is overrated. I can never live my life the "normal" way. Just because I can never be like the other kids, doesn't mean that I'm not happy. It doesn't mean that I can't smile, that I cannot laugh, that I cannot live every moment the way it should be lived. I will never be normal but that is okay with me. I am just as happy, I am just as free, and I have just as much of a life as the other kids.

I don't have to look at them with envy anymore because I know that I have my own life to live. I am fifteen and I have such a long life ahead of me.

Someday I will fall in love.
Someday I will get my own job.
Someday I will get to follow my dreams and become a writer.
Every day I will be me.

I have an issue with people who say I am different in any way. I know that I am, obviously. I know that I can never be like the other kids. I know that there will always be a school dance I have to miss because I have had surgery. I know that there will never be an easy day – a day where I don't have to fight just to get out of bed.

I know that for me, that will never happen. I will always be sick. Even though I am sick, I will still live just as much as anyone you've ever met.

A disease may take my time, it may take my body, but it will never take my mind.

It will never take my friends or the good times and it will never take away my choice. I have made my choice. I choose to live, to dance no matter what joints are dislocated, I choose to laugh although I may have a rib subluxate, I choose to go to school although it hurts my head.

This life is a choice and we each have our own. I choose to use my life to the fullest. This life is my gift. No disease can take my life away from me. When I die, I want people to say that I lived my life, smiled, and had fun despite the surgeries and pain. When I die I want to know I didn't watch my life pass me by and I took the chances I was given to live each and every moment. I will never live a life defined by normality.

WRITTEN BY MOLLY JONES

Molly Jones, age 15 is affected by Ehlers-Danlos Syndrome, dysautonomia, neuroinflammation, ACTH deficiency, RSD/CRPS, and anticardiolipin antibodies. Despite all of this, she has a love for life and likes to live life to the fullest. She has a keen interest in making a difference for others and being a positive role model. She enjoys writing, mock trial, and sciences.

Learn more at **http://www.SweetLemonPies.com**

> *"I have a problem when people say something's real or not real or normal or abnormal. The meaning of those words for me is very personal and subjective. I've always been confused and never had a clear-cut understanding of the meaning of those kinds of words." –Tim Burton*

Reappearing

They placed a hospital band on my wrist, and I blurred. Pushed into an MRI, I faded a bit more. The doctor diagnosed me and I vanished. When did you stop seeing me? When did they? As if on cue, my world closed in around me and all that remained were sterile walls and white coats. My body, a prison detached from the world, became a place of doubt and fear.

That's the thing about illness, it becomes all about you. But, here's the thing: it's not about you; it's about so much more. It took a trip to Oregon and one very special morning in the redwood forest, to remind me of the following:

I am nothing but a small part of such a great big world.

If I could find my courage to get out in that world and document what I see, maybe, just maybe, I would reappear. So, with a camera in hand, I took my first step away from illness, away from fear and walked bravely into the unknown.

It was early, when our car pulled up to the most majestic Redwood I'd ever seen. Mother Nature was performing her morning routine. Colors changed in the sky as dawn approached. That day, she wrapped the Earth in turquoise blue and wore white clouds like jewelry. As if she needed to adorn herself to impress. I grew calm in her presence. She showed off and her strength empowered me, beckoning me forward. My inner voice sounded a warning. "What if my body started to fall apart and I was in the middle of nowhere? What if I couldn't walk the trail, even for five minutes? What ifs." Pesky little thoughts that encourage fear and stagnation.

The sun came out. The birds sang. I heard water along its own journey winding through the soil. I took a breath. I felt small but safe. With my camera in hand, I am calm. I'm reappearing. It was slow at first – just a smile, maybe it was a grin. But, it did happen. I grew into focus. I flew in on the wing of a butterfly, in the beat of water dancing on rocks, and on the face of a loved one walking close beside me.

With instincts returning and a warm wind carrying me, I let go of plans made long ago… before that hospital band, before my diagnosis. Pain, like an old familiar friend, remains present, but is no longer feared. My body may have betrayed me but it will no longer define me. I discovered an entire new world with my camera; one more healing than any hospital room… One I may have never seen had I not been given this body, this illness, and this path.

"I discovered an entire new world with my camera; one more healing than any hospital room… One I may have

never seen had I not been given this body, this illness, this path." -Alyson Salzedo-Benison

WRITTEN BY ALYSON SALZEDO-BENISON

Licensed Mental Health Therapist, State of Florida. Alyson is now disabled due to Ehlers-Danlos Syndrome and Chiari malformation.

She is an avid writer and photographer.

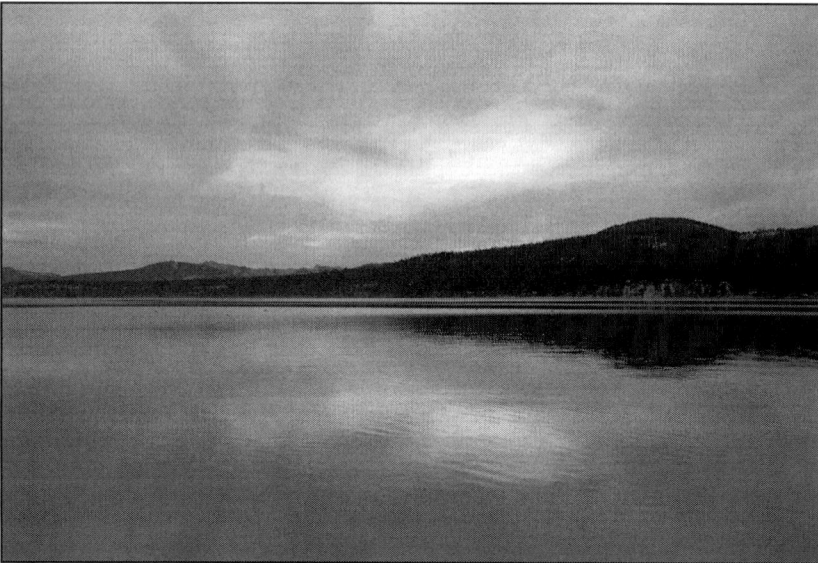

Did I offer peace today? Did I bring a smile to someone's face? Did I say words of healing? Did I let go of anger and resentment? Did I forgive? Did I love? These are real questions. I must trust that the little bit of love that I sow now will bear many fruits, here in this world and the life to come. - Henri Nouwen

Lucky To Be Alive

My story begins at an early age. I was a very active child, playing sports and overall outside activity. When I was the age of 5 I started playing softball. As I played more, I started to have more injuries, such as dislocating my thumb when playing back-catcher or twisting my ankle running. This was all chalked up to be normal, including the "growing pains."

As the years passed, I began to see doctors for high arch pain, knee pains, chest pains, back pains, and pain in most of my joints. After seeing multiple doctors, they came to the same conclusion: I was growing quickly and I wanted attention. The pain was all made up and in my head. Through my adolescent years, I bruised easily and suffered from anxiety. I was always the skinniest kid, tall but skinny and I had a huge appetite due to the high metabolism.

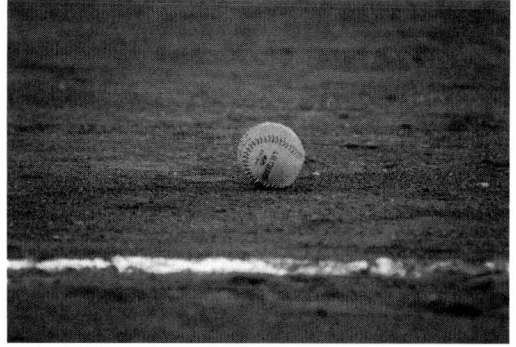

During those years, I struggled with depression. I was always in pain and my anxiety was difficult to deal with. There was nobody that understood what I was going through. The pain started to get worse and the chest pain became more frequent. As my teen years were closing and I entered my 20s, I continued to be active both in work and play. I worked long hours in construction and any free time I had I played sports. In the summer I played on 3 slow-pitch teams, a fastball team, golf, tennis, and racquetball and in the winter I played ice hockey, indoor floor hockey, basketball, volleyball, and indoor slow-pitch.

As I reached my mid-twenties, I remained active in a variety of sports and started a family. I had more problems with dislocating joints, especially my shoulders. The dislocations weren't as bothersome as the intense chest pain and coughing up blood. Each time this happened, I would see a doctor, either my GP or by visiting a clinic. I was told time and time again that I had just pulled a muscle and I was too young and healthy to have heart problems. The heart has no nerve endings, so that couldn't be the cause of my pain. This continued for another 5 years or so before my health took a turn for the worse.

In 2003, I was playing in a floor hockey tournament and I was unable to play any longer than 30-60 second shifts without coughing up blood. Although I was on the schedule to play in the tournament in October, I bowed out, knowing something was wrong.

In December 2003, I had this indescribable chest pain with intensity I had never before experienced. My wife made me go to the hospital. I was ushered into the emergency room where an ultrasound revealed a severe mitral valve prolapse. I was admitted immediately.

The cardiologist on staff that night explained to me that there was no thump-thump of a normal heartbeat, only a whooshing sound. He looked at me after hearing how active I was in sports and said, "I am amazed you are still alive." This began a two-month journey in and out of the hospital with surgery to repair my mitral valve and had a Dura-ring placed for my enlarged aorta. I saw a genetics specialist who diagnosed me with Ehlers-Danlos Syndrome and told me then that if I had not been so active I would not have had these issues.

It's now been 11 years since that life-changing moment. I do have two other valves that have started to leak and some other issues with reflux and brain fog. The combination of it all has forced me to make a career change. Even though I have health issues that are concerning, I still play some slow-pitch softball and have been in the Volunteer Fire Service for 7½ years.

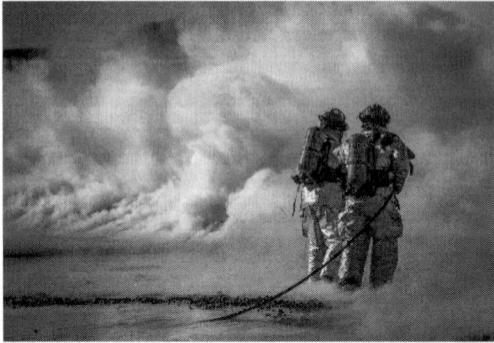

One of my greatest inspirations is my children. I have one daughter and two sons. My daughter did not inherit EDS from me, but both of my sons have. My boys have scoliosis/kyphosis and mitral valve prolapses. As I think about my journey, I want them to know that they, too, can fight with the right support of family, friends, and the support groups out there for all of us living with EDS. All of my children know that they must be their greatest advocate for their health, because no matter how much education a doctor has, they know their bodies' better than anyone else. If one doctor isn't willing to listen and investigate further, they need to rely on their support system to find a doctor who will care.

We all must stay strong and rely on the strength of our loved ones and our herd. The Zebra herd goes a long way to make living with all the issues that come with EDS much easier.

WRITTEN BY TREVOR PETERS

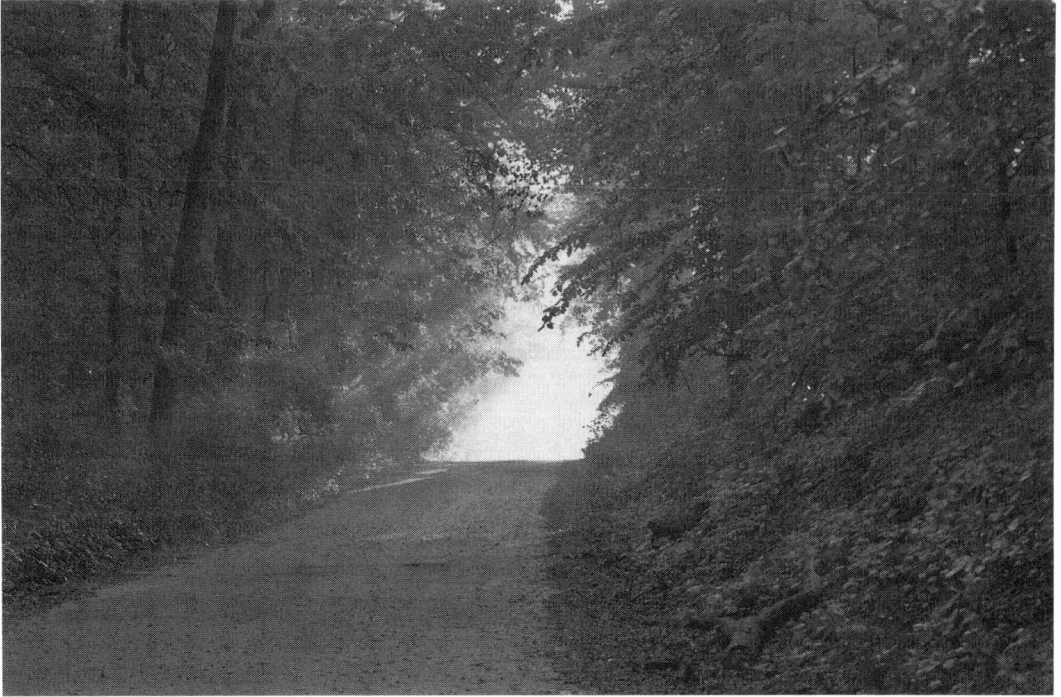

"Good humor is a tonic for mind and body. It is the best antidote for anxiety and depression. It is a business asset. It attracts and keeps friends. It lightens human burdens. It is the direct route to serenity and contentment." – Grenville Kleiser

FINAL THOUGHTS

Words... they are one of the greatest blessings that we have in our lives only when fueled by emotion that is, somehow, captured within them. Words reflect our experiences, both good and bad. They provide a means to healing and growth, friendship, and knowledge.

In some ways, words not spoken are alluring. They are pieces of lives left in the shadows... Lurking. Struggles wrought with powerful emotion that inhibits the manner in which a person lives their life. These are the moments when it is not only necessary to wield a sword, but to fight gallantly for the life that we are destined to live... Your life and mine.

There is so much more to living than to be consumed by the struggles we may face. There is opportunity to encourage, support, and give to others while focusing on what control we have within the chaos of pain, despair, and insecurity. Because living with an invisible illness brings each of those things into our lives – almost with purpose to destroy the dreams we hold deep within our hearts.

It is not without struggle to see just how we each inhibit, limit, and sabotage ourselves. But it is within that very same struggle that we are able to break through the demons, monsters, and negative self-talk that brings us to our knees.

Excuses. We have them. We either live them or annihilate them. Sometimes we do both. We make excuses for our lives because of a condition that causes pain, dislocations, or one of the many other symptoms. We can baby ourselves and pretend that choosing to sit out from a walk or spend all day in bed is okay– "Because I have Ehlers-Danlos Syndrome." At the end of the day, those excuses are detrimental to ourselves, our lives, and our dreams. We, you and me, have something incredible to give to this world. The question is: are we willing?

Are we willing to work through the physical pain to achieve something better than what is in this very moment? Are we willing to put one foot in front of the other and show this world just how incredible we are? Are we willing to take a risk of leaving behind the world of excuses for one incredible experience?

Our Stories of Strength™ would not be here if we, individually and together, entertained the excuses, challenges, or fears of the unknown. This book and the impact each individual story has made on the people who wrote them and every person who reads them are fueled by our passion to help others see just how great they are – and we are incredible.

The following timeline was written by Mysti from her perspective with edits and additions from Kendra.

June 2014

I received a message from Kendra on Twitter. She happened across my book, *Journey to Health: A Holistic Approach to Ehlers-Danlos Syndrome*, prior to attending the EDNF Conference in Houston, Texas. We conversed online – sharing of our lives, living with EDS, and raising families of our own. Those conversations turned to phone calls where an idea was born of a collection of "good news" stories coming together.

We each felt it was not only necessary, but that it was an injustice to the community as a whole, not to share these stories of strength, determination, and perseverance, while guiding others to begin shifting their perception of living to see the successes amidst the challenges. It is imperative to see the greatness that resides within each person as they step along this journey filled with countless ups and downs, celebrations and disappointments, good days and bad. We each have these moments, and often, they cloud our perception of what we are capable of achieving.

We would like to share with you a brief overview of some of what transpired during the creation of this book. The details contained here are only what Kendra and I feel can be shared publicly of our personal experiences.

July 2014

After Kendra attended the EDNF conference in Houston, we began speaking more frequently with regards to the idea of a "collection of stories." We built a rough outline of what topics we would like to cover, how we would market the book, and what challenges we expected to see. It was towards the end of July when we opted to enjoy what was left of summer with our families and pick up again in September, after school was in session and routines established. Our deadline was to release the book by May 2015, just in time for EDS Awareness Month and for Kendra's second-annual *EDS Ride for A Cause*.

August - October 2014

August came and went quickly. We laughed, played, and created memories with those nearest to us. The school year started and we settled into new routines with business, family, and school. By the end of September, talks were back in full force and an action plan was developed. Step-by-step, we began building this idea into reality. As we were finding a great workflow between us, I had an unexpected health issue with my thoracic spine. Sitting for any length of time became problematic, and progress slowed. As that injury began to heal, I was able to tackle more on my list of steps and we began moving closer to announcing our project to the world. While I was picking up momentum, Kendra attended the

EDNF Physicians Conference and came home with more passion and drive for this book to be completed. By the end of October, we were prepared to launch; however, Kendra was plagued with a systemic autoimmune reaction from the flu shot that flared complications from mast cell activation syndrome and Hashimoto's hypothyroidism.

November 2014

On November 4, 2014, we launched Our Stories of Strength™ Facebook page and announced that we were accepting submissions for the *Living with Ehlers-Danlos Syndrome* anthology. We were both working with determination as Kendra continued to fight systemic mast cell issues coupled with her thyroid not being adequately controlled. This resulted in a full-blown fibromyalgia and CFS/ME flare. We would laugh and say, "This IS really what it's about. THIS is life with EDS." Then, thirteen days after launching, I had a pop at the base of my skull that caused me to temporarily lose vision. When my vision returned, it was doubled. Doctors, neck braces, and medication consumed my world and Kendra fought through her flare to stay active on social media while I battled with insurance to have much-needed tests approved.

December 2014

In December, insurance finally approved the much-needed MRIs so my neurosurgeon could better assist my care. After scheduling those tests, Kendra and I discussed how these health challenges could pose an issue with our May deadline. Kendra focused on regaining her health and spending time with her family while I did the same. We stayed in touch and continued building upon our action plan, confident that I would, with a proper diagnosis and treatment, be able to jump back in after the first of the year.

January 2015

The days turned into weeks and before we knew it, January was here. I still had unanswered health questions, a burning desire to bring this book forward, and I walked by faith in my decision to close my Web design business so I could invest my quality working hours into Our SOS Media, LLC. As January came to a close, I had multiple diagnoses and a treatment plan to begin rehabilitating my neck with the promise of greater stability and function. While my health issues were finding the light of day, Kendra's primary business was hit as she lost her biggest client and over half of her income. The uncertainty was devastating, but we agreed that the *Living with Ehlers-Danlos Syndrome* anthology would not be our only book. We dug in with both feet firmly planted on the ground and launched our official website on January 30, 2015.

February 2015

I placed my health as my highest priority. I knew that building muscle and strengthening my neck, shoulders, and upper back was imperative for my stamina and ability to work. As I was gaining ground, Kendra fell on ice and broke her tailbone. Near the same time as her injury, she learned that her husband was facing the worst quarter of his career - and the reality of not being able to make ends meet. Kendra focused on what she could do to help provide stability for her family and I cheered her on by investing my experience into redesigning MediterinaMedicalSolutions.com, creating an EDS blog, SFHEDS.com, and outlined changes for the relaunch of EDS Patient Solutions' website. During this time, we continued working with writers and their submissions, while ironing out business details pertaining to Our SOS Media, LLC.

March 2015

It suddenly felt as though Our Stories of Strength™ was taking off. Simultaneously, Kendra and I were both facing the reality that we might need to find jobs outside of our homes. As part of my income is dependent upon the oil industry, the weight of the low oil prices became of great concern. If employment outside of my home was necessary, I knew it would be highly unlikely that I would be able to push my body in the manner necessary to continue forward with this book. Kendra's husband, who works in medical sales, received confirmation that his income would be greatly reduced due to the worst quarter of his career. As Kendra and I discussed our options, weighed the needs of our families, and what we both felt with regards to Our Stories of Strength™; we came to a conclusion: now was the time to work harder, dig deeper, and build our business with a more solid foundation to ensure it would be here for years to come. We knew the challenges we would each face physically as we spent more time working and less time exercising, but even before we could begin to see those effects, Kendra was reminded of just what EDS can do when the piercing in her ear tore through her lobe - leaving the lobe split open. Almost daily, it was as though our bodies were fighting back through increasing issues... Numbness and tingling on Kendra's face stemming from craniocervical instability as a result of sitting too much at a computer desk each day and worsening vision due to the same cause for me. A devastating EDS issue? No. We saw it as a simple reminder of how our bodies are made and why we exercise diligently. We had to believe that there was a greater purpose in all that we were going through while in the midst of putting together such an important project. By the end of March, Kendra and I had spent so much time communicating via text, email, and phone; we began to speak in symbols and single word statements that only we could understand.

April 2014

As April sprung into our lives, something incredible happened with Our Stories of Strength™ - momentum grew rapidly! Social media posts were shared, submissions came in quickly, and many people within the community reached out offering their gratitude for the book and their assistance in a multitude of ways.

We were reminded that perseverance and faith brought us to this point, as with each obstacle we faced in our personal lives and in business this project could have easily been set aside.

Our SOS Media, LLC was officially incorporated and we continued moving forward with our heads down, focused on our first major deadline. We maintained faith that this was just the beginning of something far greater than we initially anticipated. We were able to connect with people from a variety of organizations and across the world all with one mutual goal: to bring Our Stories of Strength™ to the public. As April came to a close, we were both reminded, again, what it is like to live with EDS. Kendra had a significant mast cell/EDS-related reaction, which caused her left eye to swell and bulge and her fifth strep infection since January. It was only a few days later when I dislocated my shoulder chopping chicken and had to have it reduced in the emergency room and was ordered to wear a sling for three weeks.

Throughout the last 7 months, we have both lived in messy houses with laundry piled, and once-planned meals were made on the fly and often well past our normal meal times. We have shared countless early mornings and late nights filled with accomplishing many thousands of small tasks all of which were necessary to completing this book. As we look back at the challenges we've faced and overcome, we felt compelled to share this with you as a testament of what it means to embrace living with Ehlers-Danlos Syndrome. This book, the series, and Our SOS Media, LLC were built with determination, perseverance, and strength; each quality reflective of what we, all of us, accomplish each and every day that we choose to live. The small tasks we complete each day build upon the last and show what we can accomplish individually and as a collective whole.

We hope you have enjoyed reading stories from others in this community and have found greater strength in yourself. We see these stories as a mirror of our own lives and of the lives of those we've come to know on this journey. We wanted to each offer our final thoughts to you prior to sending this off to print.

Closing thoughts from Mysti

Like many out there, my official diagnosis is relatively new. I had great hope for relief from the pain that encompassed every fiber of my being, but was met with great disappointment. I stood on the brink of ending my life and had to make the difficult decision to climb back out of that pit lined with wallowing self-pity and despair. The journey up was nothing more than small changes that built upon the last. I focused on what I could do in each moment to have a better life. In doing so, I cannot help but feel incredibly blessed by all that has changed since. In late 2013, I took control of my life and health. I learned all I could about EDS so I could change the trajectory of my life, as I knew it then. It was terrifying, difficult, and challenging in ways I had never before experienced. The hardest part, outside of finding a medical team willing to work with me, was learning how to live with EDS and not be consumed by it.

At the end of the day, no matter how my body feels, I am reminded that I have incredible power within that allows me to reach out and help others grab hold of life and make necessary changes that often seem impossible. I wouldn't be able to understand the struggle, sorrow, pain, and anguish each person feels without first experiencing all of the trials in my own life – abuse, the death of my first-born son, losing everything I once deemed important, forced to let go of a career I loved, fighting for proper care of my children, learning how to navigate and advocate within the healthcare system, losing myself in marriage, and rediscovering who I am by changing my life. Each of these challenges offered two core blessings: compassion for those facing seemingly insurmountable situations and the passion to show others that life is indeed a beautiful masterpiece and they are the artist who determines the colors that fill their world.

Where compassion and passion meet, I have been overjoyed to work on this book as the beginning foundation of Our SOS Media, LLC. Each experience of my life, personally and professionally, has led to this point. With one small detail out of place, I might not have had the perseverance to continue beyond the challenges I have faced.

It is seemingly only in retrospect where we can see the strength we've shown in life and what that means along the journey. For me, the last seven months have been wrought with challenges that reach beyond my physical health, yet I chose to focus on what I could do each day to make this life of mine, this business, and the world a bit better… Now, I stand in awe at what I have endured and overcome, my faith that God would provide, and the example of what determination means for business – for all people, even those of us living with Ehlers-Danlos Syndrome.

Closing thoughts from Kendra

In the last four years, I've been through moving my family and renovating a house just after giving birth to my third child; much of which was done by myself. I've had a disastrous medical complication due to one medication that caused toxicity and changed my life forever. I've been through a financial disaster, my marriage nearly fell apart, the worst EDS spiral I've ever been through, struggles with friends and family, more financial issues, career stressors, and the never-ending roller coaster of being in sales, health issues with my children, more personal health issues, and I was left humbled, at rock bottom, with nowhere to go but up. I have had to rebuild with no safety net and little to cling to, other than faith that all things happen for a reason and I will find the purpose in all of this.

Growing up, we did not discuss issues that you live with, because doing so was viewed as a complaining, attention seeking, or weakness. I have had to find my own answers, fight to be understood, and stand my ground when I felt that I was not heard. Most of the time, I was right: *it was not all in my head.* I have learned that there are many things I can do to prevent what I call "The EDS Spiral" and that I need to be proactive in order to protect my body and my overall health.

The truth is, many people are uncomfortable talking about something that is challenging (i.e. a chronic health condition, marital problems, etc.) or sad, because the problem is invisible, hard to relate to, or difficult to understand. People internalize what you are going through and then look at how your situation may relate to their life; thus, they become uncomfortable and scared. Some cope by looking the other way or pretending that it is not *that* bad and ignore potential issues, especially when you look "healthy." Others do not want to associate with someone who they now view as "broken." Family members may not want to admit that someone that they love has to deal with challenges, because it can often be too painful.

Personally, I do not feel sick or ill, nor do I identify myself this way. To me, being sick or ill is having something I can't live with. I do live with EDS and its comorbidities, challenges included. Living with EDS is far from easy and oftentimes it is quite humbling; especially when the reality of EDS jumps out to surprise me when I least expect it. I wake up each day, choosing to focus on the positive, because things can *always* be worse. I distract myself from the physical and emotional pain of living with EDS and the comorbidities and corresponding crises by diving into helping others. I think, in many ways, helping others has helped me face my own trust issues and believe it has made me stronger. An added bonus is that volunteering provides me an outlet to discuss living with EDS, as I seldom speak about challenges I face with those around me, nor do they ask. My focus is on being supportive for other people versus needing help myself. Being in a vulnerable position resulted in great emotional pain, feelings of loneliness, and trust issues due to relationship challenges with some people who were closest to me - all feelings that I hope to help others avoid.

I would not be who I am today, have met the people I have, or been so blessed with so many opportunities to help others – including this anthology – without receiving my diagnosis of Ehlers-Danlos Syndrome. I have become comfortable with who I am without concern for what those around me think. There's nothing to prove with regards to my health and everything to gain by discussing Ehlers-Danlos Syndrome publicly to educate, advocate, and change the perceptions of how others view this condition within the community and outside, too.

How could I truly help those with EDS, if I was hiding such a huge part of my life and who I am? For every one person close to me who may be uncomfortable, I have been able to help five people view their life with EDS differently. Many have found hope, determination, and the strength to persevere; yet, I saw myself as still needing to do the same. The more involved I am, the more opportunities arise for me to help make a difference in peoples' lives. Meeting and working with so many incredible people has provided me strength to keep going and confirmation that the way I've approached my life with EDS is not off base. However, the journey over the past year of putting this anthology together has changed what I once perceived as insecurities into confidence in who I am and what I am doing. For that, I am forever grateful.

What I have come to realize is that I have a strength that I never knew I had; one true strength that empowers me through helping and making a difference in the lives of others, while traveling my own journey. We really are stronger together.

RESOURCES

Suicide Hotline
1-800-273-8255

Ehlers-Danlos National Foundation
http://ednf.org

EDS 2016 International Symposium
http://eds2016.org/

EDS Awareness
http://chronicpainpartners.com

Ehlers-Danlos Syndrome Network Cares
http://www.ehlersdanlosnetwork.org/

EDS Today
http://edstoday.org/

Center for Ehlers-Danlos Syndrome Alliance
https://www.cedsa.org/

Life as a Zebra Foundation
http://www.zebranation.org/

EDSers United Foundation
https://www.edsers.com/

Atlantic Ehlers-Danlos Syndrome Society (Nova Scotia)
http://www.atlanticedssociety.ca/

Ehlers-Danlos Syndrome Canada
http://www.ehlers-danlossyndromecanada.org/home.htm

Ehlers-Danlos Support Group (UK)
http://www.ehlers-danlos.org/

Hypermobility Syndromes Association (HMSA)
http://hypermobility.org/

Ehlers-Danlos Syndrome (Netherlands)
http://www.ehlers-danlos.nl/site/index.cfm

Ehlers-Danlos Syndrome (Swiss)
http://www.swiss-eds.ch/

Ehlers-Danlos Syndrome (Sweden)
http://ehlers-danlos.se/

Ehlers-Danlos Syndrome (Denmark)
http://ehlersdanlos.dk/

Ehlers-Danlos Syndrome (France)
http://www.afsed.com/

Ehlers-Danlos Syndrome (Norway)
http://www.eds-foreningen.no/

Irish EDS & HMS
http://irishedsandhms.ie/

Information for Healthcare Professionals
http://strengthflexibilityhealtheds.com/eds-information-and-resources-for-healthcare-professionals/

Information resources for Patients
http://strengthflexibilityhealtheds.com/eds-information-resources-and-news-for-patients/

Blood volume testing
http://my.clevelandclinic.org/heart/services/tests/nuclear/bloodvolumetesting.aspx

Dysautonomia International
http://www.dysautonomiainternational.org

Aortic Dissection
http://www.thedoctorstv.com/videolib/init/1548

Good North American Doctors
https://www.facebook.com/groups/1438285386415297/

Good European Doctors
https://www.facebook.com/groups/372374862916395/

Good Australian Doctors
https://www.facebook.com/groups/287952358017187/

Marfan Syndrome
http://www.marfan.org/

Osteogenesis imperfecta
http://www.oif.org

Epidermolysis bullosa
http://www.debra.org/whatiseb

Stickler Syndrome
http://sticklers.org

Alport Syndrome
http://www.alportsyndrome.org/

Loeys–Dietz Syndrome
http://loeysdietz.org/

Williams Syndrome
https://williams-syndrome.org/

Cutis Laxita
http://www.merckmanuals.com/home/children-s-health-issues/hereditary-connective-tissue-disorders/cutis-laxa

Ectopia Lentis
http://www.marfan.org/ectopia-lentis-syndrome

Familial Thoracic Aneurysm and/or Dissection
http://www.marfan.org/familial-aortic-aneurysm

Fragile-X Syndrome
http://www.fragilex.org/

MASS Phenotype
http://www.marfan.org/mass-phenotype

Mitral Valve Prolapse Syndrome
http://mitralvalveprolapse.com/

WHAT IS EHLERS-DANLOS SYNDROME?

Ehlers-Danlos Syndrome (EDS) is a group of heritable connective tissue disorders that are caused by various defects in the collagen protein used to make our connective tissues and is classified as a rare disorder affecting 1:5000 people. Based upon recent research, the prevalence of EDS exceeds this number and could be as high as 1:100 to 1:200 people (Collins, 2015; Nielsen, 2013). Each type of EDS is characterized by a distinct problem in making or using one of the types of collagen. Collagen is the body's most abundant protein and can be found in nearly every component of our bodies, from our ears, to our eyes and mouth, to our heart, surrounding our internal organs and veins, connecting our joints, in our bones and down to the tips of our toes. Collagen is a strong protein that provides both strength and elasticity to our tissues, as well as allows our tissues to be stretched safely without damage or without being stretched past a normal range. Basically, Ehlers-Danlos Syndromes are structural problems caused by defects to the "glue" that holds our bodies together.

A perfect example is described on the website for the EDS 2016 International Symposium (eds2016.org).

"If one builds a house with bad materials, perhaps half [of] the necessary wood or aluminum nails, one knows there will be problems. Some problems can be anticipated, but because those materials were used everywhere and aren't necessarily visible, one may be surprised. Being built out of a protein that doesn't behave the way it should can result in widespread difficulties in a wide range of severities, even in places one wouldn't think are connected until one realizes that collagen is used there, too."

For the reasons stated above, Ehlers-Danlos Syndrome is viewed as a multi-systemic condition that presents differently in those affected. Symptoms of Ehlers-Danlos Syndrome often include, but are not limited to: joint hypermobility (This is not to be confused with flexibility as people can be hypermobile without being flexible and vice versa. Hypermobile joints are loose or unstable and slip or dislocate.); dislocations; prone to bruising easily and tissue fragility – such as skin that tears easily; vascular issues and internal organ rupture; poor wound healing; abnormal scarring; chronic fatigue; chronic pain; cardiac abnormalities; foot deformities; TMJ dysfunction; low muscle tone; hernias; early osteoarthritis and degenerative discs; various GI problems and allergies; chronic headaches; eye problems; dysautonomia and POTS; dental issues; chronic pelvic pain in women; congenital defects of the spine, including the head, neck and the entire spinal column; ADD/ADHD; learning disabilities; circulatory issues and much more. Often times, patients are diagnosed with various conditions that are considered comorbid to EDS - the presence of one or more additional disorders that can co-occur with the primary disease or disorder, such as fibromyalgia, chronic fatigue syndrome/ME, mast cell activation disorders, IBS, gastroparesis and functional GI issues, POTS and other dysautonomias, CRPS/RSD, Raynaud's and other circulatory conditions, various dermatological conditions, mitral valve prolapse and other cardiac conditions, osteogenesis imperfecta, Chiari malformation, scoliosis, craniocervical instability, tethered cord syndrome and other structural congenital conditions of the spinal column, osteoarthritis and degenerative disc disease, migraines and other types of chronic headaches; and various conditions of the eye, ears, and skin.

Pain can be widespread—for instance, collagen makes up the fascia, which is the tissue sheet that holds everything together and wraps around the entire body— but the pain may not show up in MRIs or X-rays, and will be probably be out-of-proportion to any findings.

Currently, there are 6 major types of Ehlers-Danlos Syndrome, including vascular Type, which is considered most severe due to the increased risk of arterial, cerebral, and organ rupture at any age. The 6 main types of EDS are:

- Hypermobility Type
- Classical Type
- Vascular Type
- Kyphoscoliosis Type
- Arthrochalasia Type
- Dermatosparaxis Type

However, additional types of Ehlers-Danlos Syndrome are being discovered as more research is done and our understanding increases. Additional types of EDS are:

- Musculo-contractural type
- Multiplex congenital
- Periodontitis Type
- Progeroid
- B3GALT6 Deficiency
- Cardiac valvular
- FKBP14-related
- Spondylocheirodysplastic
- Tenascin-X Deficient
- Periventricular heterotopia, ED variant

Other types mentioned in literature, but do not have a clear definition, are disputed, or have been reclassified include:

- Classic-like EDS
- Beasley-Cohen
- Friedman-Harrod Type
- EDS/OI Overlap
- Vascular-like
- Dermatosparaxis
- Type)
- RIN2-Syndrome
- EDS Type V (X-linked - found in one family)
- Occipital Horn Syndrome (EDS Type IX)
- Brittle Cornea Syndrome
- EDS Type X (Fibronectin Deficient - found in one family)
- The EDS Type XI (Familial Joint Hypermobility Syndrome - may be linked to Hypermobility type)

Ehlers-Danlos Syndrome is usually diagnosed based upon the Beighton Score; a nine point clinical assessment for joint hypermobility. Those that score greater than a 4/9 are diagnosed with EDS Hypermobility Type. However, this assessment often discounts people who have various other signs and symptoms of EDS, because many score lower on the Beighton Score. In that case, The Brighton Diagnostic Criteria is used and includes major and minor criteria for diagnosis. Many times, people have overlapping symptoms over different types of EDS, including vascular type and a genetic test either through blood sample or skin biopsy is warranted in order to give a definitive diagnosis; however, a genetic test is not a current requirement to receive an EDS diagnosis.

Despite being named in the early 1900s, it is quite obvious that EDS is far from rare and that both men and women of every race and ethnicity can inherit it. Many have suggested that EDS may be one of the most prevalent, yet under-diagnosed disorders. Currently, there is no cure. However, many symptoms can be prevented or treated as they arise and individuals can lead healthy, active, and fulfilling lives.

Ehlers-Danlos Syndrome often has signs and symptoms that overlap with other heritable connective tissue disorders. There are over two hundred distinct heritable disorders of the connective tissue and approximately thirty-six have overlapping features. Many times, one or more heritable connective tissue disorders can part of broader condition, such as EDS. Below are a few examples of other heritable connective tissue disorders:

- Marfan Syndrome
- Peyronie's disease
- Osteogenesis imperfecta

- Epidermolysis bullosa
- Stickler Syndrome
- Alport Syndrome
- Congenital Contractural Arachnodactyly
- Loeys–Dietz Syndrome
- Williams Syndrome
- Cutis Laxita
- Ectopia Lentis
- Familial Thoracic Aneurysm and/or Dissection
- Fragile-X Syndrome
- MACS Syndrome (Macrocephaly, Alopecia, Cutis Laxa and Scoliosis)
- MASS Phenotype
- Mitral Valve Prolapse Syndrome

To help distinguish heritable connective tissue disorders from autoimmune connective tissue disease, we have included a brief summary.

Autoimmune connective tissue diseases may have both genetic and environmental causes. Often, they are also referred to as systemic autoimmune diseases. Genetic factors may create a predisposition towards developing these conditions. They are characterized as a group by the presence of spontaneous overactivity or underactivity of the immune system. In response to a substance the body believes is unwelcomed, antibodies are produced and instead of attacking the trigger, they attack the body's own tissues. In the event of underactivity, the body is unable to fight against infection. The classic collagen vascular diseases have a "classic" presentation with typical findings that doctors can recognize during an examination and through a blood test. There are numerous people who have both a heritable connective tissue disorder, as well as an autoimmune connective tissue disease. Autoimmune connective tissue diseases that fall under the classic collagen vascular diseases umbrella include:

- Systemic Lupus Erythematosus
- Rheumatoid Arthritis
- Scleroderma
- Sjögren's Syndrome
- Mixed Connective Tissue Disease
- Psoriatic Arthritis

WHAT IS THE ZEBRA?

"When you hear the sound of hooves, think horses, not zebras."

This is a phrase that is referred to often when medical students are in medical school and the term "zebra" is used in reference to a rare disease or condition. Doctors are taught to expect common conditions, versus incorrectly diagnosing patients with rare conditions.

However, we know that "Zebras" DO exist. And because of this, obtaining a proper diagnosis and treatment can be more difficult when the condition you have is considered rare, yet in truth is rarely diagnosed, patients are often misdiagnosed. The identity associated with a Medical Zebra was adopted in order to bring our community together.

It has been suggested that we are not Medical Zebras, but horses of many different colors, instead.

The following stems from a presentation by Dr. Heidi A. Collins in reference to horses. "A horse of a different color metaphorically represents something that may be completely separate from what one originally expected. Frequently, a horse of a different color may be a complete surprise, an unexpected truth or a feature that seems somehow out of place. ~Idioms Unpacked"

ABOUT KENDRA NEILSEN MYLES

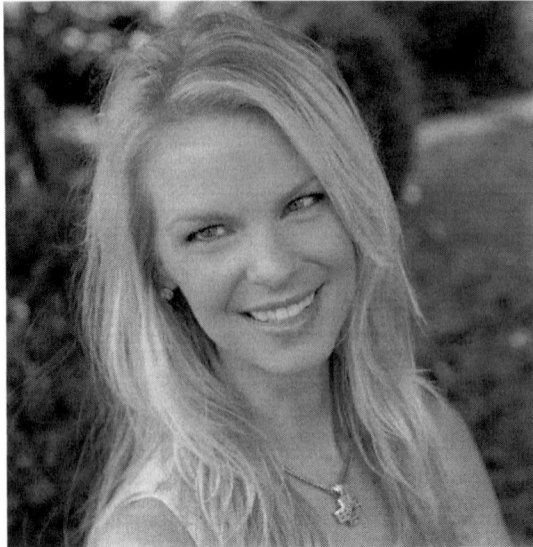

Kendra Neilsen Myles holds a B.S. in Public Health with a concentration in exercise science from University of Maryland. After working with health education programs at Columbia Hospital for Women in Washington, DC; sports medicine/physical therapy programs including Fitness for Health in Rockville, MD; and at the Women's Health Clinic at University of Maryland while she was in college; Kendra opted to put continuing her medical education on hold, in order to help care for her mother who was sick with breast cancer. She found the "job of her dreams," working for Johnson & Johnson as a territory manager for their Ortho-McNeil Women's Healthcare division. Kendra remained in her position for 6 years, earning numerous top sales awards during her tenure, until she was diagnosed with Ehlers-Danlos Syndrome after the birth of her first child. Using the year and half that she had to take off from her career with Johnson & Johnson, she focused on regaining her strength and determination through ways that she knew were best to care for herself, with the goal of returning to work in the profession she loved. During this time, Kendra sought a means to support her family through self-employment. Once her employer benefits ended, Kendra was required to apply for social security disability and after 2 denials, she was awarded benefits at the age of 27. Faced with a difficult decision, Kendra made a bold choice and declined the benefits of Social Security Disability and immediately started Mediterina Medical Solutions. Kendra believed she could build a business that would meet her health and financial needs – and Mediterina Medical Solutions, almost a decade later, proves this to be true as she has sold a fantastic product to hospitals through exclusive rights in the Washington D.C. and Baltimore, MD area.

Over the last 8½ years, Kendra has been an independent medical representative for Histoacryl Tissue Adhesive, grown Mediterina Medical Solutions into more than "just something" she could do on her own, and provided life-changing freedom for herself and her family. Along with providing resources and support for Histoacryl and other medical device and supply products, Kendra started a small photography business with her sister called, SistersMedia.

Kendra has spoken about Ehlers-Danlos Syndrome from a patient's perspective several times to the first-year medical students through the Department of Genetics at the University of Maryland and for the last 2½ years, she has served as a volunteer for the Ehlers-Danlos National Foundation by answering HelpLine emails. It was through Kendra's personal experience as a patient with EDS seeking information and resources where she saw voids that needed to be filled due to a lack of awareness and knowledge. Her desire to help people with EDS, personal passion for fitness, health, and nutrition, coupled with the knowledge that her healthy lifestyle was the main reason why she has been able to maintain a normal life despite living with several chronic health conditions, was what prompted her to start EDS Patient Solutions 4 years ago.

Kendra believes consistency, discipline, and hard work pays off in her personal and business lives. Due to these beliefs, she opted to focus on the growth of Mediterina Medical Solutions, volunteering with EDNF, supporting the EDS community through various activities, and her health following her most recent EDS spiral following back-to-back pregnancies, instead of diving into the development of EDS Patient Solutions right away.

In marrying her active lifestyle with her passion to aid the EDS community, Kendra organized *Ride for a Cause* benefitting The Ehlers-Danlos National Foundation (EDNF) at Zengo Cycle. This was the first "active" fundraiser for EDS ever done in the US and was just one of the ways that Kendra has been able to help serve the EDS Community, while also sharing how passionate she is about living a healthy and active lifestyle with EDS.

It was through Kendra's desire to find others with EDS like her and her need to recruit for the EDS *Ride for a Cause*, she networked on her Instagram profile, Strength/Flexibility/Health/EDS, and branched-out to other social media platforms. Through recruiting for the EDNF fundraiser, she was able to further see how imperative an active and healthy lifestyle was to overall quality of life for everyone living with EDS. Subsequently, Kendra was provided the opportunity to share this information with the teens at the 2014 EDNF conference in Houston, Texas. Her passion was ignited with greater intensity and she found a clear direction of what she wanted to do. During this time, Kendra discovered with whom she wanted to work; which led to the official launch of EDS Patient Solutions.

Through connecting with others on Kendra's personal health, fitness, and "living with EDS" account, which included Mysti, the author of *Journey to Health: A Holistic Approach to Ehlers-Danlos Syndrome* and mom of 2 boys her own boys' ages, it was more that apparent 2 things needed to happen immediately:

1. SFHEDS needed a website/blog

2. Together with Mysti, a platform for patients was needed to provide the opportunity to share good news stories as they live with chronic illnesses. Those stories, published collectively, would begin with an anthology called, *Our Stories of Strength™ - Living with Ehlers-Danlos Syndrome*.

Our Stories of Strength™ series is just the beginning of a long-standing partnership between Kendra and Mysti.

As SFHEDS's blog approached completion, *Our Stories of Strength - Living with Ehlers-Danlos Syndrome* by Our SOS Media, LLC sent for print, the 2nd Annual EDS *Ride for a Cause* benefitting EDNF will be held late May 2015, additional opportunities came to partner with healthcare professionals who are interested in learning more about diagnosing, treating, and caring for patients with Ehlers-Danlos Syndrome. These opportunities include partnering with two local physical therapists that have a shared interest in helping the EDS population beginning in spring 2015, and additional EDS related projects with others in the community.

It is through of all these recent life developments and new opportunities that EDS Patient Solutions and Our SOS Media, LLC have the opportunity to provide others with knowledge and tools necessary to regain their strength, health, and life while living with Ehlers-Danlos Syndrome and other chronic conditions through health and life coaching, support services, and networking with healthcare professionals.

Kendra lives in Bethesda, MD and is the owner of two small businesses, Mediterina Medical Solutions and EDS Patient Solutions, as well as is the Co-Owner of Our SOS Media, LLC. Kendra writes for her blog, strength/flexibility/health/EDS, continues to speak about EDS through various opportunities, and is also a volunteer with The Ehlers-Danlos National Foundation (EDNF). She has been married for 12 years and has 3 beautiful children. Other than having a passion for fitness, health, and nutrition; Kendra is a closet Apple genius, avid first-adopter of all things health and fitness-tech related, photographer, traveler, reader and thoroughly enjoys helping others.

You can connect with Kendra through <u>Facebook</u>, <u>Instagram,</u> on <u>Pinterest</u> and on Twitter at <u>@SFHEDS</u> and <u>@KNMyles</u> or visit <u>sfheds.com</u> for the latest on living a healthy and active life with EDS.

Professional photographs by Heather Owens. PhotosByHeatherOwens.com

ABOUT MYSTI REUTLINGER

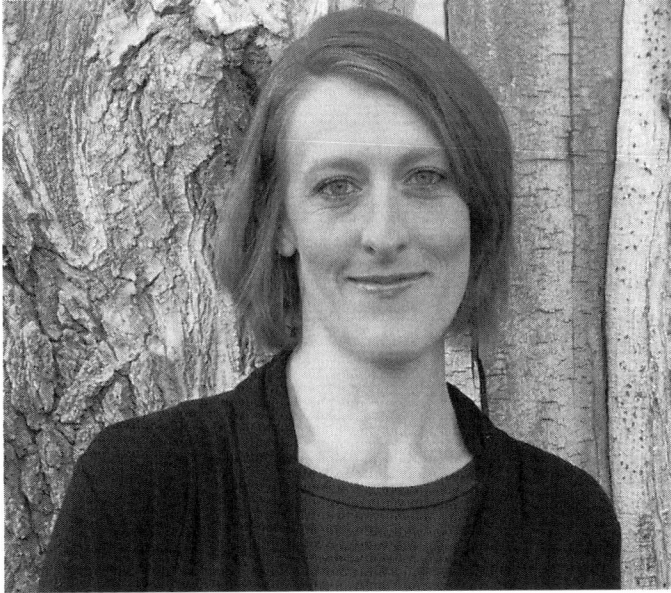

Mysti Reutlinger has a long history of working with small and medium businesses as a Web designer, content editor, and consultant. In her consulting role, Mysti has had the pleasure of educating businesses on harnessing multiple income avenues online to generate additional income; capitalizing on their established presence and mission. Outside of business-to-business work, Mysti Reutlinger has worked with public figures, actors, movie directors, and musicians to create a socially unified mission for their private and not-for-profit ventures.

In 2010, Mysti Reutlinger turned down her first publisher's contract in lieu of self-publication. Her book, *The Pantry Cleaner: Chemical Free Cleaning* was released in February 2011 and has since sold over 30,000 digital and print copies. In early 2013, Mysti was requested to teach a course to grieving parents based off her own experiences after losing her firstborn son 13 years prior. Mysti's course was based on the art of practicing gratitude and was well received. Numerous parents attending the course requested a journal that followed the same premise. On August 11, 2013, Mysti released her second book, *A Gratitude Journal for Grieving Parents* as a result. Just under a year later, *Journey to Health: A Holistic Approach to Ehlers-Danlos Syndrome* was released, capturing the seemingly insurmountable, debilitating, and devastatingly depressing Ehlers-Danlos spiral that lead to her diagnosis as well as her determined journey to regain her health.

Mysti studied psychology at the University of Wyoming while gaining extensive knowledge as a restaurant and bar manager. She acquired national certifications and led multiple training and development courses in the art of sales, food handling, and customer service. She appreciates the knowledge gained and how it applies to her work within the bereavement, chronic illness, and business sectors.

In 2008, Mysti gave birth to her youngest son at 24-weeks in gestation. During their journey through the NICU, PICU, and multiple hospital visits, she learned how to be the best advocate for her son's care while actively researching to understand the health issues faced to adequately communicate with physicians. Following her son's last extended hospitalization in 2009, she began aiding parents of preemies by teaching them how to advocate for their children and themselves through one-on-one consultations via phone. As her son has aged, Mysti has found herself in a position to help parents with visually impaired children find new, exciting ways to educate and engage them in the world.

Through the publication and marketing of *Journey to Health: A Holistic Approach to Ehlers-Danlos Syndrome* Mysti met Kendra Neilsen Myles and a friendship developed around the joint desire to live well. Amid countless conversations, the duo had an inspired idea for a series of books that would inspire others living with chronic illnesses and Our Stories of Strength™ by Our SOS Media, LLC was formed.

When Mysti isn't designing a website, implementing advertising strategies, writing, editing, giving her time to help those in need, or planning her homesteading adventure; she can be found playing with her children, dancing in the rain, and photographing the beauty in the world.

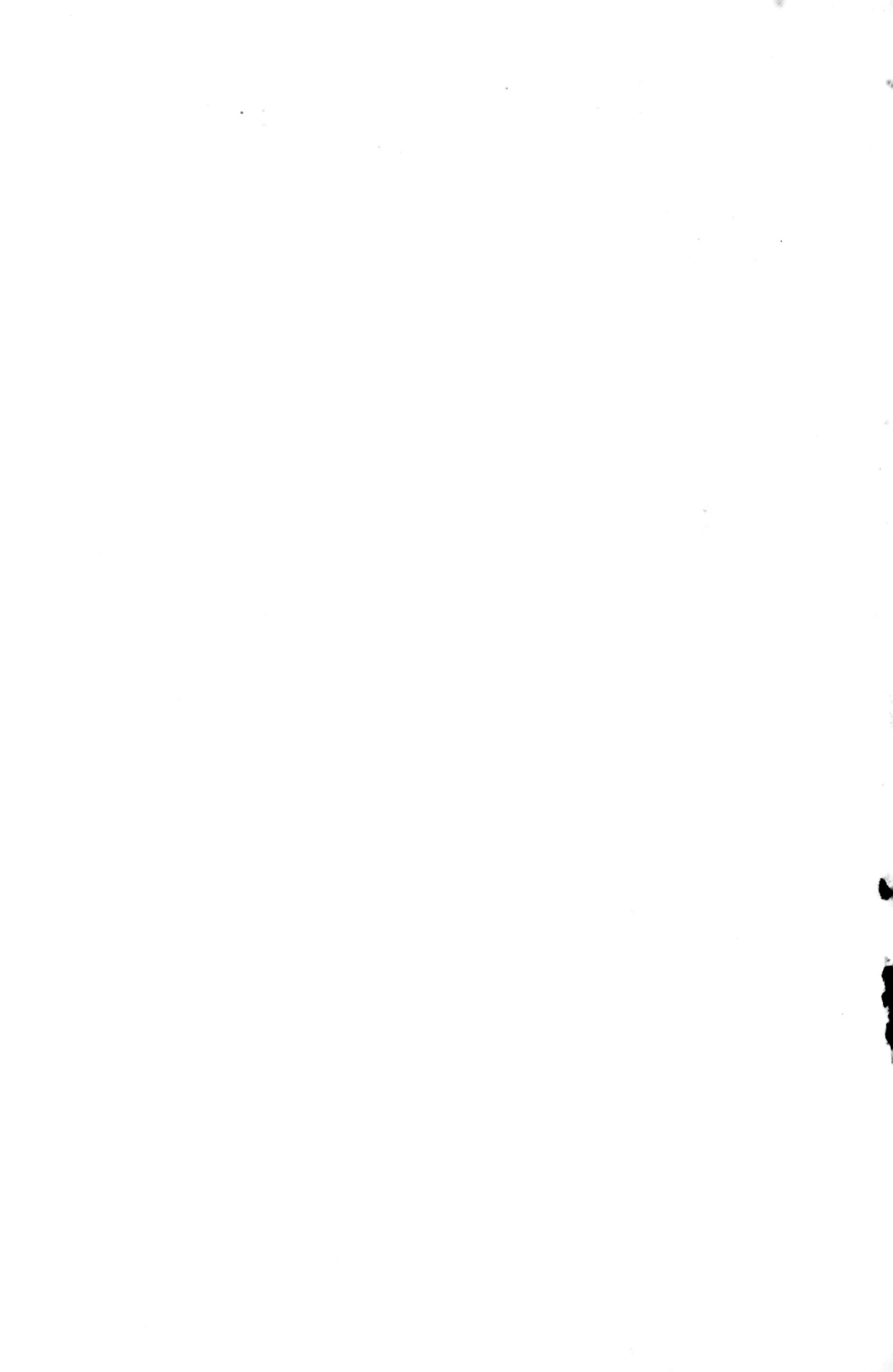

11208152R00123

Printed in Great Britain
by Amazon.co.uk, Ltd.,
Marston Gate.